Ischemic Stroke

Edited by Pratap Sanchetee

Published in London, United Kingdom

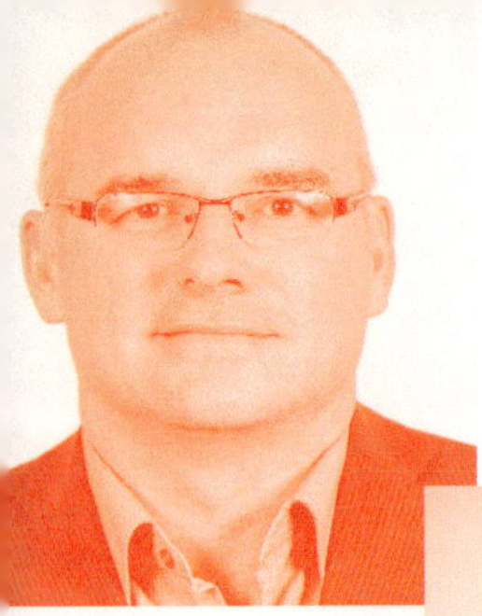
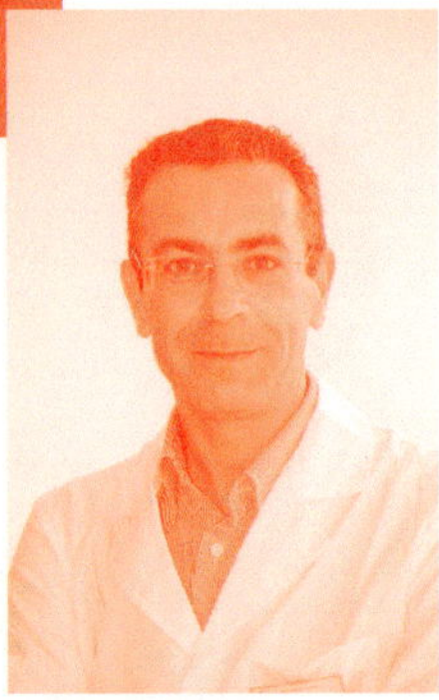
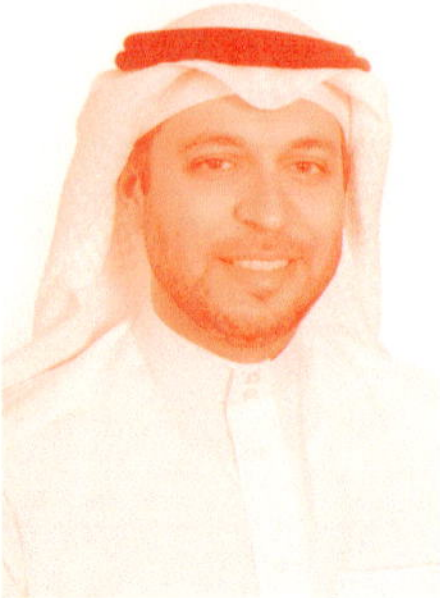
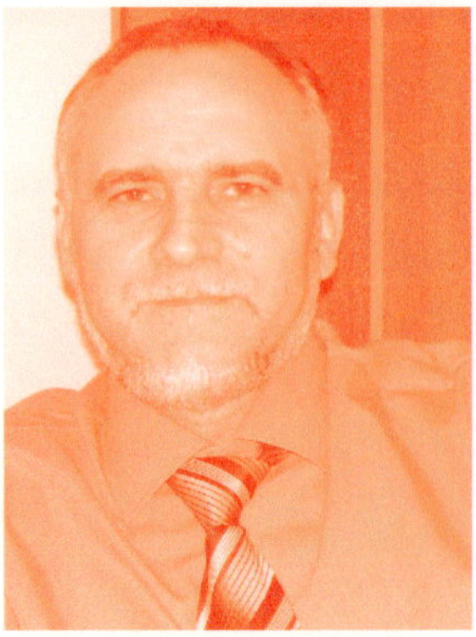
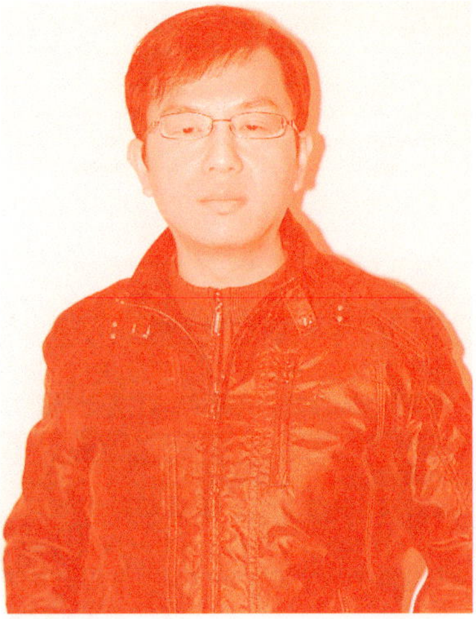
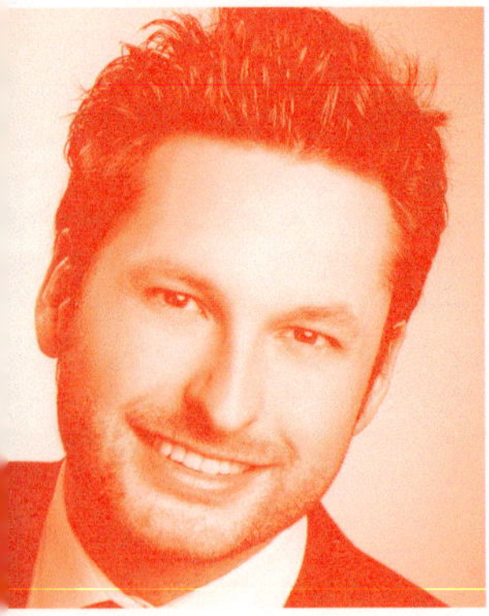
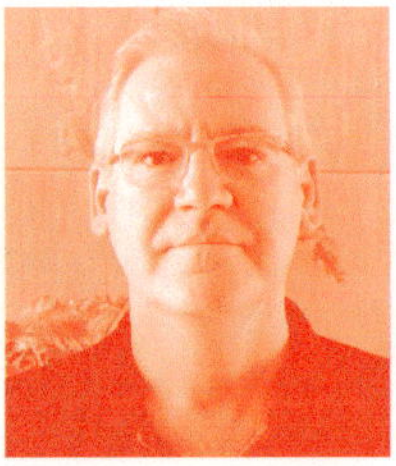

IntechOpen

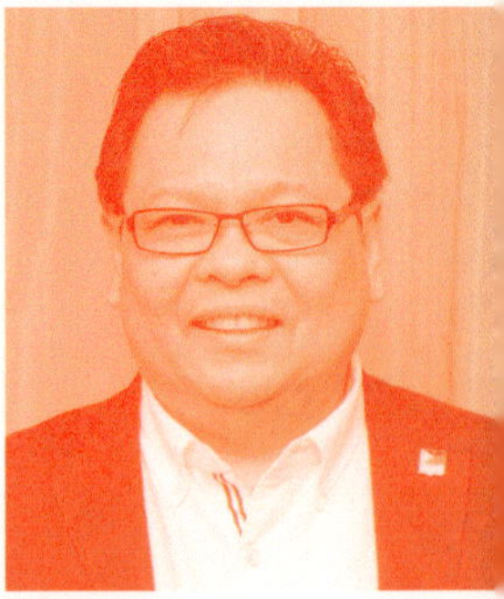
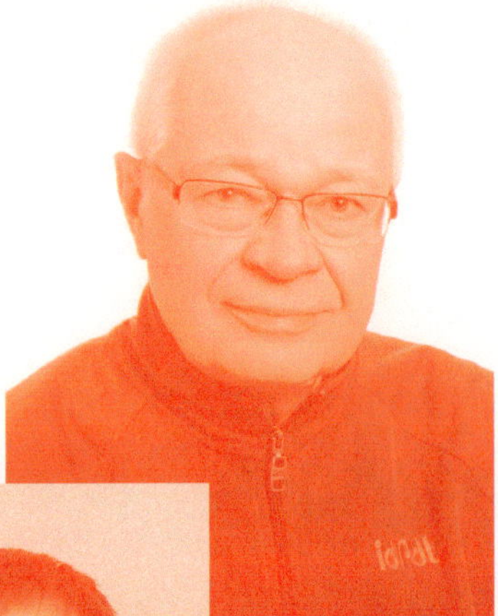
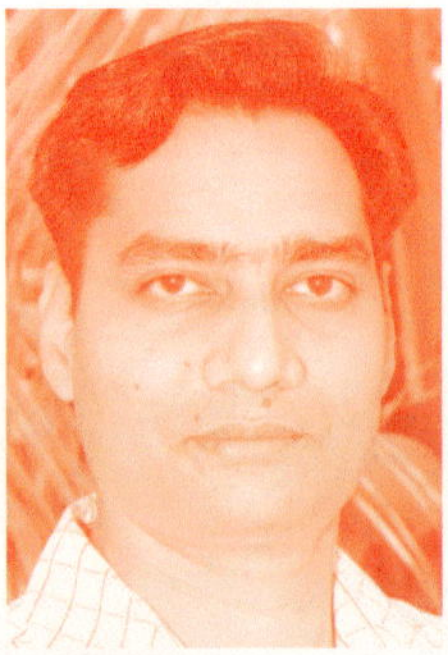
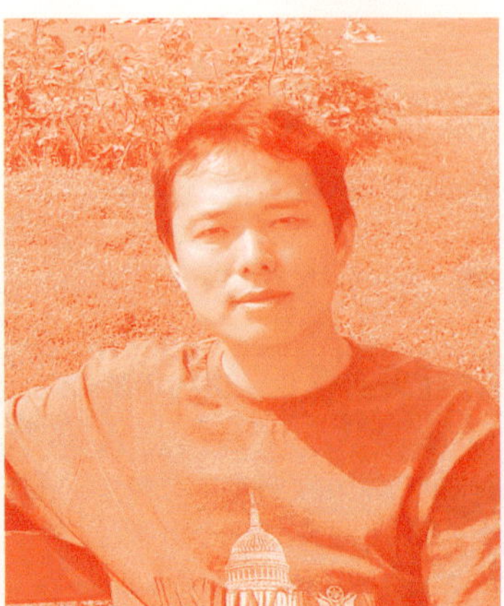
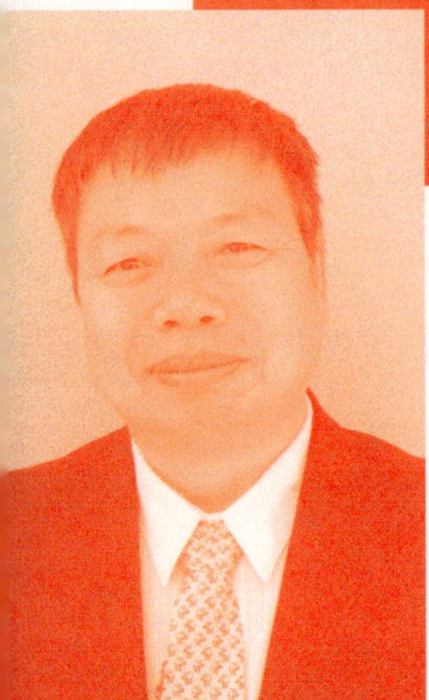
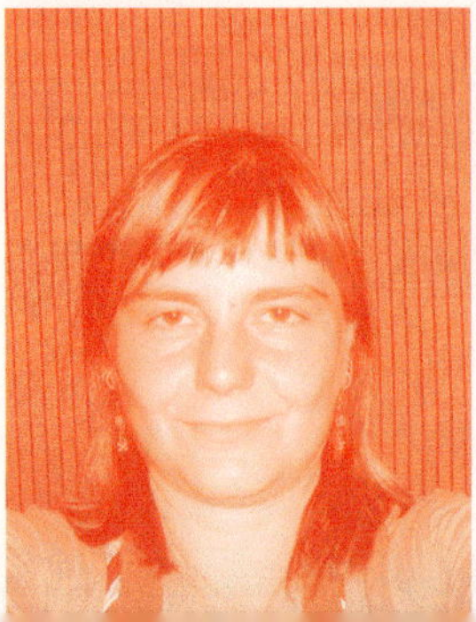

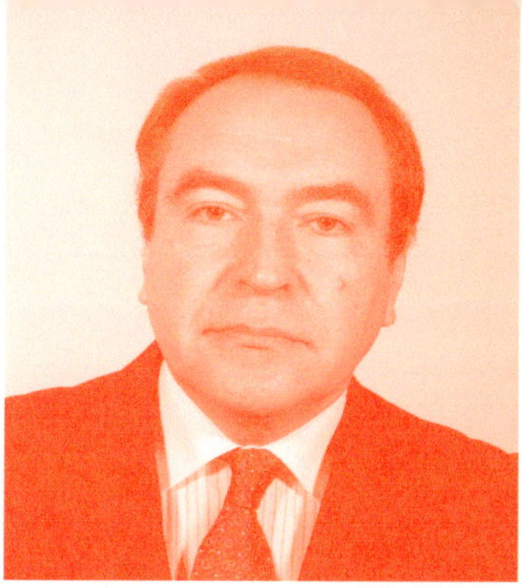

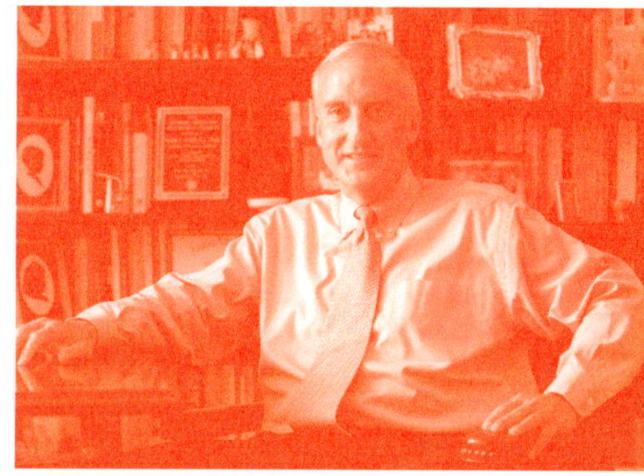

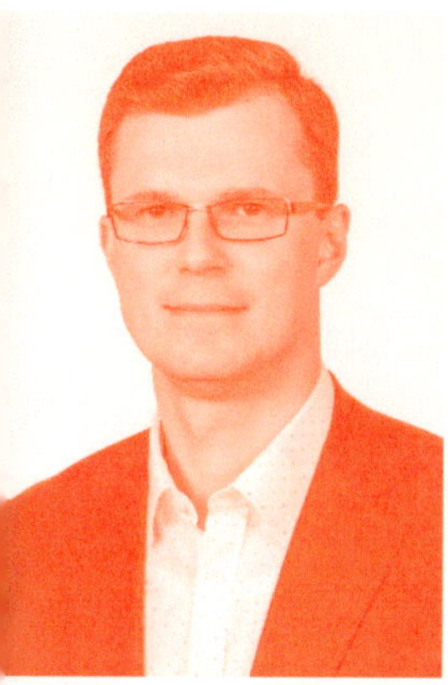

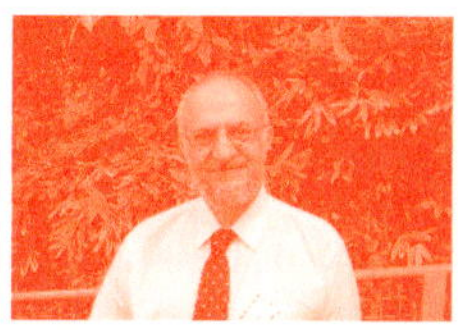

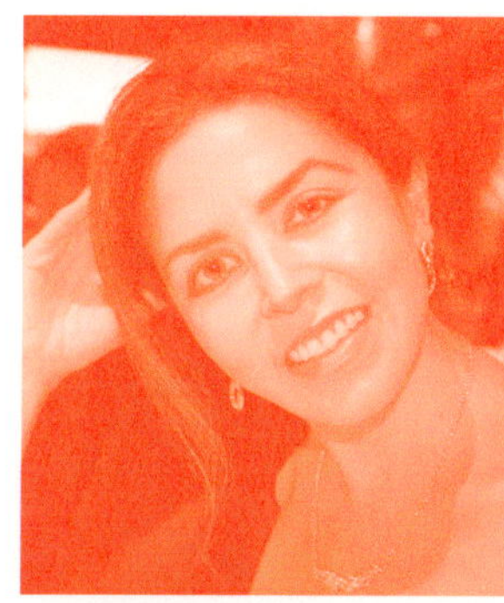

Supporting open minds since 2005

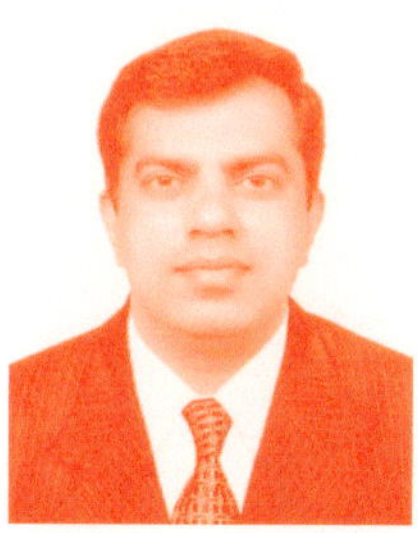

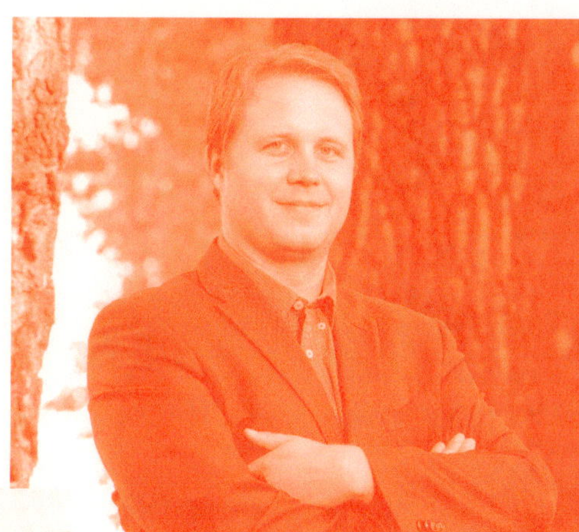

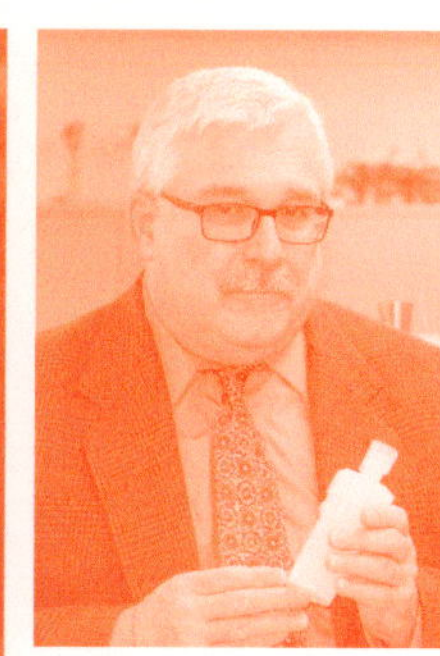

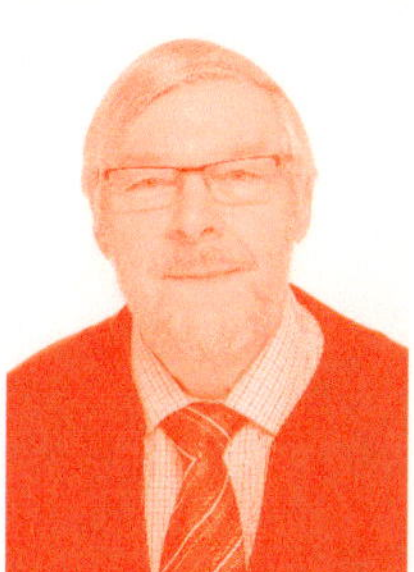

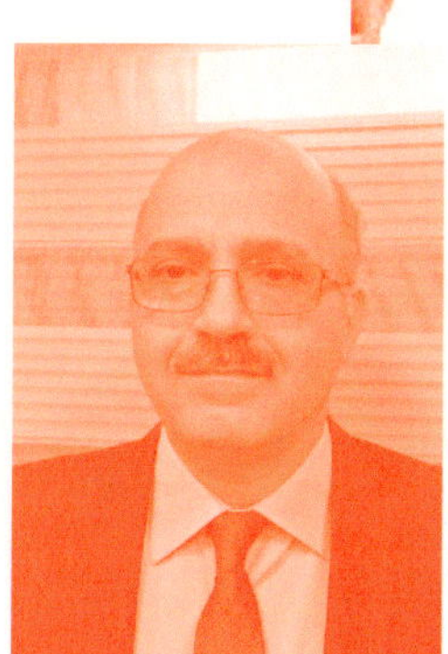

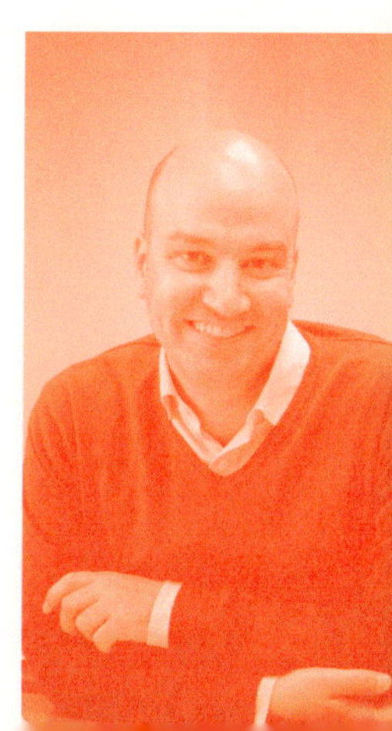

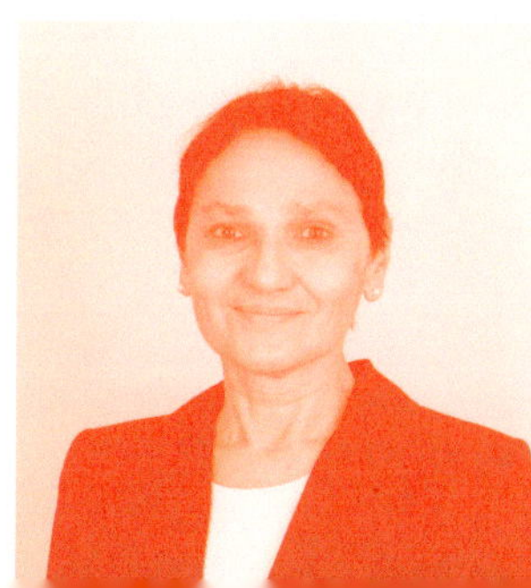

Ischemic Stroke
http://dx.doi.org/10.5772/intechopen.86623
Edited by Pratap Sanchetee

Contributors
Hayder M. Al-kuraishy, Irina Alexandrovna Savvina, Anna Olegovna Petrova, Carmen Adella Sirbu, Diana Mihai, Cristina Florentina Plesa, Any Docu Axelerad, Alice Elena Munteanu, Claudia Minerva Ghinescu, Dragos Catalin Jianu, Silviana Nina Jianu, Ligia Petrica, Traian Flavius Dan, Georgiana Munteanu, Aliza Brown, Krishna Nalleballe, Rohan Sharma, Nidhi Kapoor, Karthika Veerapaneni, Sisira Yadala, Sanjeeva Onteddu, Vasuki Dandu, Madhu Jasti, Suman Siddamreddy, Pratap Sanchetee, Ali I. Al-Gareeb

First published in London, United Kingdom, 2021 by IntechOpen
IntechOpen is the global imprint of INTECHOPEN LIMITED, registered in England and Wales, registration number: 11086078, 5 Princes Gate Court, London, SW7 2QJ, United Kingdom
Printed in Croatia

British Library Cataloguing-in-Publication Data
A catalogue record for this book is available from the British Library

Additional hard and PDF copies can be obtained from orders@intechopen.com

Ischemic Stroke
Edited by Pratap Sanchetee
p. cm.
Print ISBN 978-1-83962-394-3
Online ISBN 978-1-83962-395-0
eBook (PDF) ISBN 978-1-83962-396-7

For EU product safety concerns:
IN TECH d.o.o., Prolaz Marije Krucifikse Kozulić 3, 51000 Rijeka, Croatia, info@intechopen.com or visit our website at intechopen.com.

Meet the editor

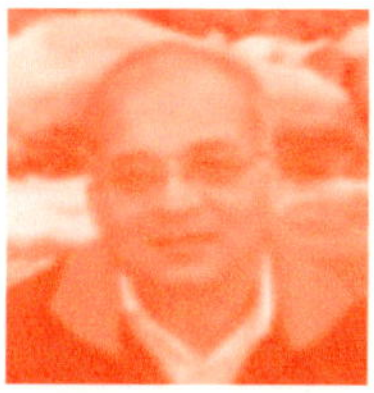

Dr. Pratap Sanchetee is a first batch alumnus of Dr. SN Medical College, Jodhpur, and achieved his MBBS in 1970. Subsequently, he received his MD diploma (Medicine) from the University of Rajasthan in 1974, and DM (Neurology) from the Postgraduate Institute of Medical Education & Research (PGIMER), Chandigarh in 1985. He served in the Armed Forces India as a Physician and Neurologist for 24 years and retired as Lt Col in 1998. From 1994 to 1998, he also served as an Associate Professor, Armed Forces Medical College, Pune. He was awarded Chief of Army Staff's Commendation in 1980. Since 1998, he has been pursuing clinical practice in neurology at various hospitals at Jodhpur and at Guwahati Assam. He has been a Visiting Professor, Ph.D. guide, and advisor to Jain Visva Bharti University (JVBI) and Bhagwan Mahaveer International Research Centre (BMIRC), Ladnun, Rajasthan since 2009. He is a Director of Research at the Spiritual Training Research Foundation (STRF), Mumbai, India. His areas of active interest are the mind as an interface between soul and body, meditation and the brain, and delivery of neurology care in society. Dr. Sanchetee has a life membership of 9 national associations. He is the editor of four books and has published 110 original papers, chapters, and review articles in national and international journals. He is currently the Chairperson of the "Tropical Neurology Subsection" of the Indian Academy of Neurology. He regularly participates in national and international conferences and presents academic papers. He was an executive editor of the Medical Journal Armed Forces India and Journal of Indian Academy of Geriatrics.

Contents

Preface

Stroke continues to be a major public health issue. It is the third leading cause of death and disability across the globe. Its early identification, early treatment, and prevention are major issues that confront a treating physician. Early recognition of the disease involves public awareness, an emergency transport system, a good and well-rehearsed stroke care program, and an organized rehabilitation setup both at the hospital and in the community. We have understood the importance of early intervention and the quote 'time is brain' has been understood by neurologists across the globe and by most physicians. Our endeavor now should be directed to the public at large and paramedics in particular. Until recently, a stroke was considered to be an illness of old people but we are diagnosing an increasing number of such cases in young people. Carmen et al. in their article on ischemic strokes in young people have dealt with this issue in detail. Aphasia and difficulty in swallowing, though an important component of stroke-related disabilities have not been stressed in detail in current textbooks. Cătălin et al. in their article on vascular aphasia have elaborated on this problem.

Although a stroke is a common condition, the availability of a neurologist or stroke specialist is quite scarce. Today, management of a suspected case of stroke is done by a specialist team of medical and paramedical personnel who are trained and tuned to act swiftly without wasting any time. However, the availability of such facilities is limited by cost and geographical distance. To deal with and manage it in the periphery, telestroke is a novel concept. Through this, many patients now have the access to a qualified stroke specialist in remote areas. Aliza et al. in their article 'Telestroke: A New Paradigm ' have highlighted its application.

Advances in imaging, newer therapeutic agents, and endovascular management have revolutionized the management of ischemic stroke. Intravenous thrombolysis in a window period of four and half hours is a revolutionary development and now it is possible to salvage the ischemic brain and save many patients from death and gross disabilities. Irina et al. have reviewed many burning issues related to managing ischemic strokes and have given us some practical tips. Protection of brain tissue from ischemic damage during various phases i.e. pre-hospital phase, during hospitalization, and poststroke phase, is a long-felt need. Unfortunately, none of the available agents or procedures have been proved clinically and this has been highlighted in the last article.

Currently, we are witnessing a new era in the management of strokes and I am hopeful that continued research will get us to a satisfactory solution. This book along with another book from IntechOpen titled 'Ischemic Stroke of Brain' is a great source for postgraduate medical students in medicine and neurology who have an interest in stroke care.

Dr. Pratap Sanchetee, MD, DM (Neurology)
Consultant Neurologist,
Sanchetee Neurology Research Institute,
Rajasthan, India

Section 1

Ischemic Stroke - Diagnosis

Chapter 1

Current Trends in Stroke Rehabilitation

Pratap Sanchetee

Abstract

Stroke remains a leading cause of adult disability. The social, physical and psychological consequences of stroke are devastating. With better understanding of causation and breakthrough advances in management, we are witnessing a greater population of stroke survivors with varying neurological and functional deficits. Poststroke rehabilitation is a multi-disciplinary and multi-modal endeavor and not a 'one size fits all' intervention. A combination of interventions may be better suited to treat motor and sensory impairments, cognitive problems and psychological issues. There is great interest in exploring novel rehabilitation technologies to augment conventional therapies to reduce neurological disability and improve function. Yoga and spirituality, though ancient practices, are finding a bigger role in field of rehabilitation. In spite of good potentials for recovery, these rehabilitative measures are underutilized and major barriers are limited availability, geographical distance, high cost and lack of awareness about its benefits. While conventional measures are well engraved, this article review the recent concepts in stroke rehabilitation.

Keywords: gait rehabilitation, repetitive task training, mirror therapy, cognitive rehabilitation, robotic therapy, telerehabilitation, virtual reality, yoga, meditation, spirituality

1. Introduction

Stroke is a major public health concern and remains a leading cause of adult disability [1, 2]. The social, physical and psychological consequences of stroke are devastating. In spite of best treatment available, 30–50% stroke survivors are left with significant physical and/or psychological disabilities and consequent decline in quality of life (QOL) [3]. Such patients require long-term rehabilitation to the restore and improve motor functions for the paralyzed limbs. There is marked inconsistencies in quality of care and rehabilitation services across the globe.

The rehabilitation of the stroke is a multidisciplinary process involving doctors, nurses, physiotherapist, occupational therapists, neuropsychologists, linguistic and speech specialists, audiologists, and nutritionists [4]. With better understanding of causation and breakthrough advances in management, we are now witnessing a greater population of stroke survivors with varying neurological and functional deficits [5, 6]. There is great interest in exploring novel technologies to augment conventional therapies to reduce neurological disability and improve function.

2. Prognosis in stroke recovery

Approximately one third to half of the patients is left with significant physical and/or psychological disabilities [4, 5]. This leads to a marked decline in QOL which increases with passage of time. Neurorehabilitation with conventional physiotherapy, occupational therapy and speech therapy offers them a good opportunity to regain QOL and activities of daily livings (ADLs). A large number of prognostic factors have been identified [2, 7]. Extent and severity of initial injury to brain is perhaps the most important factor for stroke recovery. Many techniques are available to assess which include bedside evaluation, functional magnetic resonance imaging (fMRI) and transcranial magnetic stimulation (TMS) etc. [5, 7]. It has also been observed that presence of comorbid conditions such as past stroke or transient ischemic attacks, diabetes, hypertension, dyslipidemia, cardio-respiratory status, advancing age, and degree of periventricular white matter hyperintensities on MRI adversely affect outcomes [5].

3. Physical therapy

While motor deficit and spasticity management is well organized, there is a requirement to develop a holistic module considering other deficits such as difficulty in swallowing, nutrition, fear of falls, sensory impairment, dysarthria, aphasia, cognitive impairment and depression also.

3.1 Muscle strengthening and early Mobilization

Strength training is defined as an intervention where participant exercised a muscle or group of muscles against an external resistance. Both active and passive exercises are safe to perform for hemiplegic stroke patients and can induce functional improvement [8]. Passive exercises, by the therapist or with motorized ergometer, are defined as movement of the body without the effort of the patient. Progressive resistance exercises are functional patterns of movements against progressively increased resistance or weight. Passive and active muscle movements and progressive resistance training is most commonly employed and perhaps most effective therapy to improve motor power and functions including walking, gait and balance [9]. They are also effective in reduction of fatigue and improvement in QOL in individuals with stroke. Most of stroke patients have a high prevalence of cardiovascular risk factors that are potentially modifiable with exercise. However, to document such quality of improvement, high-quality methodological designed studies are required.

It has been observed that passive exercises over limbs and early mobilization even during acute stage of stroke leads to better recovery [5, 10, 11]. Apart from psychological benefit, early mobilization also enhances neuroplasticity. Thus acute rehabilitation can be recommended on a continuous basis once cardio-respiratory status is stabilized.

3.2 Repetitive task training (RTT)

It is based on the principle that our brain is tuned for complexity and pattern of task rather than just on a single movement. Repeated practice of task-specific motor activities (e.g. lifting a cup) on regular basis is more effective than simple movements at joints. In RTT, an active motor sequence of a desired movement is performed repetitively within a single training session, aimed toward a clear functional goal. There is low to moderate quality evidence for RTT in improving upper and lower limb functions, walking and functional ambulation up to six months post treatment [12].

3.3 Constraint-induced movement therapy (CIMT)

CIMT involves constraining of the non-paretic arm while doing task-oriented training with paretic limb. It was developed mainly to upper limb functions and perhaps is the most investigated intervention in stroke rehabilitation [13]. Original CIMT include constraining of non-paretic upper limb with a sling or glove for 90% of the waking hours 2 weeks, while affected limb undergoes intensive training of the 5–6 hours per day. In modified version of CIMT (mCIMT), the therapy sessions are less intense (1/2 hour to 2 hour per day for 3 days a week) and have better tolerance and acceptability [14]. Both CIMT and mCIMT have demonstrated benefits in motor function, arm-hand activities, and ADLs on immediate as well as on long-term follow-up [13, 14].

3.4 Mirror therapy

In mirror therapy, a mirror is placed in the person's midsagittal plane reflecting movements of the non-paretic side as if it were the affected side [15]. It is provided for 15–60 minutes three to seven times a week for four to eight weeks. A sustained mild to moderate improvement in motor function, motor impairment and ADLs has been observed mainly with upper limb after mirror therapy which maintained for 6 months or more [12, 15, 16]. However, there was a small to insignificant improvement in pain and visuospatial neglect. One of the additional advantages with mirror therapy is that it can be performed even in presence of severe or complete paralysis of a limb [16]. Thus it can be safely employed as an adjunct for training post-stroke impairments (motor, sensory, perceptual deficits) in acute, sub-acute, and chronic phases.

3.5 Botulinum toxin

Poststroke spasticity is seen in approximately a quarter of patients which interfere with ADLs, personal hygiene, social participation, and QOL [17]. Effective spasticity management is often challenging for the clinician as commonly prescribed drugs to treat spasticity such as lioresal, tizanidine, benzodiazepines, and dantrolene sodium have limited role [18]. Botulinum toxin A (BoNT-A), one of the most potent biological toxins, is extensively used now a day to treat focal spasticity [18]. Injection BoNT-A combined with conventional rehabilitation training is a major advance in improving motor functions [17]. It safely and effectively reduces the muscle tone and increases the range of motion. The major disadvantage with this form of therapy is that its effect vanishes in 2–6 months and it requires skill person to administer it. Though experience is limited, it is perceived that functional outcome of many patients would be improved if BoNT-A is introduced aggressively.

3.6 Gait rehabilitation

Improvement in walking capacity is one of the main concerns with stroke victims and their family. Marked limping with unsteady gait and poor obstacle clearing increases the risk of falling [19]. Thus strengthening of trunk and hip muscles (particularly hip extensor) and gait training are major goals in rehabilitation [20]. Six-min walking test is a simple assessment of gait in community setting.

Common available techniques for gait training are walking stick, stationary cycle, stepping machine and treadmill training with or without support [21]. Gait training with robotic-assisted therapy and augmented or virtual reality (VR) is now being evaluated and preliminary results are encouraging [20]. In VR, treadmill training is supplemented with visual cues through projectors that display shapes on the walking surface. The training schedule includes specific exercises for gait symmetry, coordination enhancement and gait agility. A daily session of 30-min duration for 4 weeks has provided a significant improvement in gait speed and in balance [20].

4. Rehabilitation technologies

Though conventional motor rehabilitation are effective, the major limitation with them is an inadequate dose of rehabilitation therapy, in terms of repetition and intensity [22]. Rehabilitation technologies are defined as 'those whose primary purpose is to maintain or improve an individual's functioning and independence, to facilitate participation and to enhance overall well-being'. Such devices are quite helpful in engaging patient's interest and motivation. A wide range of such applications are available e.g. robotic and virtual reality technologies, assistive devices, neuroprostheses and smartphone applications.

4.1 Robotic devices & virtual reality (VR)

While robotic devices are characterized by machines capable of carrying out a series of complex actions automatically, virtual reality (VR) is characterized by a machine produced interactive simulations to allow users to engage in environments that closely resemble the real-world [22]. During such simulation, visual and multisensory feedback constitutes an important attribute. Many robotic devices and VR technologies are available which facilitate joint movements, walking, improve muscle strength, motor function and ADLs in upper limb and possibly in lower limb [22]. Electromechanical-assisted gait training combined with conventional physiotherapy is more effective than training without these devices. Combining robotic and VR technologies increase the intensity and amount of rehabilitation training. However, such devices are complex and costly for routine use and there is a requirement to develop a low cost simple module.

4.2 Electrical stimulation (ES)

Electrical stimulation (ES) is one of the most widely used therapy and its reported benefits include spasticity reductions, improvements in range of motion, improved sensation and reduced pain. In spite of promising benefits, there are insufficient evidences in case control studies [3]. However, its benefit in stroke rehabilitation has not been adequately demonstrated. There are many types of ES and commonly applied in stroke are neuromuscular electrical stimulation (NMES), functional electrical stimulation (FES) transcutaneous electrical neuromuscular stimulation (TENS) and iontophoresis (to administer medicines). Combining ES with physical exercises is critical for achieving maximum results.

NMES is delivered by surface electrodes over involved muscles and giving pulse stimulation. In 15–30 minute sessions for 4–8 weeks. FES is a technique that uses low-energy electrical pulses to induce movements in a muscle or group of weak muscles in paralytic limb. They are useful in retraining voluntary motor functions such as grasping, reaching and walking [23]. TENS is a non-invasive inexpensive and self-administered technique to relieve pain associated with stiffness and contractures in hemiplegic limbs [24]. During TENS, pulsed low intensity electrical currents are delivered through surface electrodes.

5. Regenerative therapy

Till recent, it was believed neural tissues do not regenerate. Now we have learnt that it is possible to reconstruct neural circuits with transplanted endogenous neural stem cells [25]. In many studies, stem or progenitor cells like neural stem cells, neural precursor cells, embryonic stem cells, mesenchymal stem cells, and induced pluripotent stem cells showed a beneficial effect in restoration of lost neuronal and vascular elements. Cell therapy considers not only replenishment of deficit cells but also to create a regenerative environment. Preliminary evidences suggest that regenerative cell-based therapies can lead to functional recovery in stroke patients [26].

5.1 Growth factors and neuromodulators

There are studies that higher levels of many growth factors has positive impact on stroke recovery, neuroplasticity, neurogenesis, neuronal and and dendritic changes, synaptogenesis and cortical reorganization after stroke [27]. Such factors include vascular endothelial growth factor (VEGF), hepatocyte growth factor (HGF), Brain-derived neurotrophic factor (BDNF), nerve growth factor (NGF), glial-derived thrombospondin 1 and 2, erythropoietin (EPO),and growth-inducing proteins (neuromodulin, CAP23, mArCKS). While exogenous growth factor therapy has emerged as a potential treatment for ischemic brain injury in recent years, more studies are needed to quantify timing, dosing, route of administration, optimize combination therapy and their place in clinical setting [28].

5.2 Drugs to enhance motor recovery

Recovery after stroke depends on the neuroplasticity which is defined as ability of brain to reestablish the structural and functional organization of neurovascular networks [29]. While most of studies have focused on neuroprotection in the acute phase, drugs to enhance recovery during chronic phase of stroke has not been adequately researched. Currently, there are some drugs that can facilitate brain repair and improve clinical effect even years after stroke onset. Drugs that have been evaluated for recovery after stroke in animals and poststroke patients are D-amphetamine, levodopa and other dopaminergic agents, fluoxetine, niacin, inosine, and cticoline. However, no significant clinical benefit has been observed with any of the drugs.

5.3 Cognitive rehabilitation

Cognitive impairment is perhaps second common deficit after motor impairment following stroke [6]. Though 30% of them recover spontaneously, a large number of such patients remain cognitively impaired. Cognitive rehabilitation therapy (CRT) is defined as a wide range of interventions to improve cognitive functioning by (i) reestablishing or strengthening previously learned patterns of behavior or (ii) establishing new patterns of cognitive activity or compensatory mechanisms for impaired neurological functioning [30]. There are many types of cognitive deficit in postsroke patients and they include forgetfulness, confusion, disorientation, problems with attention, executive functioning, and information processing etc. [31]. However, being subjective, it is difficult to quantify cognitive deficits and we must develop suitable biomarkers including MRI, and magneto-encephalography (MEG) to assess them. Cognitive rehabilitation is still far from satisfaction.

Cognitive deficit interact with motor deficits in exponential way to result in disablement after stroke. Thus combining motor and cognitive rehabilitation is a practical way of enhancing recovery after stroke particularly in moderate-to-severe cases. CRT is an individualized program of specific skills training and practices involving memory, attention, self-awareness, problem-solving skills, executive functions, social skills, self monitoring, activities planning and task sequencing [32]. To have complete benefit, CRT should be administered as a part of the multi-disciplinary and not as a "stand alone" approach. Right hemispheric infarct patients need additional spatial retraining to promote rapid recovery [33].

5.4 Non-invasive brain stimulation

There is a substantial reorganization in brain after stroke [34]. Non-invasive brain stimulation (NIBS) has been shown to enhance neural plasticity and is a promising strategy in cognitive and motor training. Current research is limited to a small number of cases with poor methodologies. The commonly studied NIBS techniques are transcranial direct current stimulation (tDCS) and repetitive transcranial magnetic stimulation (rTMS) [34]. Such interventions induce positive effects on force production by increasing cortical activity in the ipsilesional hemisphere and decreasing cortical activity in the contralesional hemisphere [5, 6, 35]. A good improvement has been seen with NIBS in hemispatial neglect, gait speed and performance in ADLs in poststroke patients [11].

6. Remote rehabilitation

6.1 Tele-rehabilitation

Newer technologies for rehabilitation have the limitation of cost, complexity and limited access to patients in remote or rural areas. Furthermore, limited resources prevent patients from receiving intensive treatment and extensive attention at rehabilitation centres. Telerehabilitation, also known as e-rehabilitation, is the delivery of rehabilitation services over telecommunication networks and the internet [36]. It provides access to rehabilitation services at a remote area using communication technology [14]. Apart from physical therapy, with telerehabilitation services we can deliver speech therapy, occupational therapy, audiology services and psychological support also. It is a fast growing application and has the potential to improve access and reduce treatment disparities for stroke patients who live in rural areas. Combining telerehabilitation with in-person services reduces the personal visit to rehabilitation centres.

6.2 Biofeedback and wearable sensors

Hospital or clinical based functional assessment and monitoring therapy is not only time consuming with personal bias, it lacks real life individualized situation in a familiar environment [8]. Wearable sensor technology addresses many of these limitations and offers home-based therapies which can be monitored remotely [37]. Last two decades have witnessed a significant advancement in technology and low cost miniature sensors have been developed which enable objective and long-term monitoring in a patient's habitual environment [38]. Most of sensors currently in vogue are either inertial measurement units (IMUs) or electromyography (EMG) based sensors.

Biofeedback training in rehabilitation aims to improve outcomes by educating and engaging patients [39]. This is close loop system where a person learns through the data provided by sensors placed over body or head. These data are then fed in a processor unit connected to an output motor device. Neurofeedback (NF) training is also a close loop system where a person learns by self-regulating his/her own brain activity through real-time feedback [40]. EEG alpha wave feedback has been studied extensively. Recently researchers have started using real-time functional magnetic resonance imaging (rt-fMRI) signals to modulate brain activity [41].

Conventionally subject attends 2–3 sessions per week for 4–6 weeks. A mild to moderate grade improvement has been observed in motor functions, gait control, attention, memory, concentration, reading, coordination, visual perception and emotional state in chronic stroke patients. Additional advantage of this system is that it can be used during acute stage of stroke when strenuous physical exercises are not possible. During chronic stage of stroke it facilitates neuroplasticity and functional reorganization.

6.3 Brain–computer interface

Brain–computer interface (BCI) or brain–machine interface (BMI) is an upcoming technology in stroke rehabilitation [4, 5]. Brain signals are recorded through a sensor (either surface EEG signal or an invasive microelectrodes) are transmitted a computer processor to decode it and formulate a signal for intended actions with robotic limb or wheelchair. It can also be utilized as electrostimulation devices or assist with motor imagery. This high cost venture is currently in experimental stage.

7. Yoga and spirituality for stroke rehabilitation

Yoga and Meditation: Yoga is an ancient Indian science and way of life [1, 42]. Practice of yoga consists of physical postures (*asanas*), controlled breathing (*pranayam*), body relaxation, and control of thoughts and mind (meditation). Meditation is an essential component of yoga and is now being practiced worldwide. These practices strengthen willpower and control of mind and body to work in perfect synergy [1]. They have been extensively studied for promotion of physical and mental health and in management of diverse clinical disorders [42]. They are known to promote cardio-respiratory health and to reduce stroke related risk factors (e.g. carotid atherosclerosis, dyslipidemia, hypertension, diabetes, and coronary artery disease) [43].

Spirituality: There is no agreed definition of the term spirituality. It is a blend of humanistic psychology with an individual relationship with a higher powers and the subjective experience about the "deepest values and meanings by which people live," [44, 45]. Higher levels of spirituality are known to be associated with a better QOL for stroke survivors and the caregivers [44]. To have its wider application, it is necessary to distinguish it with religion which is an institutionalized and community based doctrine, beliefs, practices and rituals [44]. It must be clarified that being spiritual does not necessarily mean religious whereas the reverse is true.

Bastille and Gill-Body and Singh et al. demonstrated that following practice of yoga and meditation there was significant improvement in muscle power and range of movements in hemiplegic limbs and some positive effects in the Berg Balance Scale (BBS), Timed Movement Battery (TMB) and quality of life (QOL) as assessed

Step Description	Duration
1. **Place & Position** (decided on patient's condition and disablement) • Select a quite place with least distraction. • Comfortably sitting on a chair or lying in the bed.	2–3 minutes
2. **Posture** (*asanas*) and loosening movements: • Based on patient's condition movements can be active, passive or assisted. • Based on physical disablement, one can increase upto 10–15 minutes	15 minutes
3. *Pranayam* (breathing exercises) and controlled breathing: • Make breathing slow, long and rhythmic. Take a deep breath in with mouth closed and hold it comfortably for 2–4 seconds. Then exhale effortlessly with mouth closed. Repeat this initially for 5 times in 2 minutes and with practice gradually increased it to 9–11 times in 7–10 min. *Pranayam* has shown to enhance body oxygen utilization, improve concentration and clean the respiratory passages.	10 minutes
4. **Body relaxation with awareness** (*Kayotsarga*) • Instruct body to relax each part, one by one, from toe to the upper part of the head. Autosuggest for relaxation of muscles, body and mind. Maintain this relaxation for 5 minutes and with practice increase it to 10 minutes.	5 minutes
5. **Meditation** • **Concentration meditation:** With eyes closed focus your attention on a single object, idea, sensation or an aspect of divinity (e.g. counting or monitoring breathing, reciting a mantra, visualizing processes in the body, external object, etc) at the exclusion of all other thoughts. Distracting thoughts will invariably appear but try to ignore them by focusing the mind through autosuggestions. • **Open mindedness:** This is a higher stage which can be practiced after one has mastered concentration meditation. Instead of focusing attention, there is expansion of awareness and attention. All sensory inputs, be it internal (thoughts, feelings, memory, etc.) or be it external (sound, smell, etc.), are perceived as they are without any prejudice and in a nonreactive way. This it provides a stimulus to gain access to knowledge, self-realization, and for soul (consciousness) purification.	10–15 minutes
6. **Conclusion** Gently close your meditation session. Rub your hands and move your body freely	One minute

Table 1.
Yoga and spiritual practices module for stroke rehabilitation.

with Stroke Impact Scale (SIS) [46, 47]. Cognitive and psychological improvement with reduction in anxiety and depression are additional advantages with mediation which is helpful for stroke patients and caregivers [48–51].

Yoga and meditation practices allow neurorehabilitaion in less complex and highly individualized environment [47, 50]. Being a low-cost model, it improves availability of rehabilitation in low- to middle-income countries also. However, yoga and meditation program should be tailored to deliver personalized interventions according to each person's profile and rehabilitation needs (time after stroke, level of impairment, function and mobility). A suggested module as designed by the author is given in **Table 1** and should be modified as per patient's need and disablement. Though these practices are effective and less labour intensive, there is a lack of evidence-based review to support the claim [44]. To have a larger acceptance by academic community, rigorous experimental studies are needed.

Mechanism of improvement: Long practice with yoga has been associated with increase gray matter density in structures involving memory, self-awareness, and compassion. fMRI studies have shown increased gray matter in hippocampus, prefrontal cortex, cingulate cortex and brain networks including the default mode network (DMN) [52]. Contrasting to this, there was decrease in volume of amygdala, associated with fear, anger and stress.

Epigenetic refers a way to regulate gene activity in real time without modifying the DNA sequence. It allows body to function with changing environment. Yoga and related practices have shown to alter gene expression particularly those related to free radicals handling, mitochondrial energy production and utilization, inflammation processes and apoptosis [53].

8. Conclusions

The field of stroke rehabilitation has a bright future. In spite of good potentials for recovery, these rehabilitative measures are underutilized and major barriers are limited availability, geographical distance, high cost and lack of awareness about its benefits. Such interventions should consider variables such as time after stroke, type and level of impairment, and functional need. In recent period, we have witnessed many novel concepts and interventions such as robot-assisted training, magnetic and electrical stimulation, brain–computer interface, telehealth, stem cells, biotherapeutics, and the use of virtual environments. Yoga and spirituality, though ancient practices, are finding a bigger role in field of rehabilitation. Medical and paramedical practioners involved in stroke care should be aware of them and educate the patients and caregivers.

Author details

Pratap Sanchetee
Sanchetee Neurology Research Institute, 429, Pal Link Road, Jodhpur 342008, Rajasthan, India

*Address all correspondence to: pratap.sanchetee@gmail.com

References

[1] Lazaridou A, Philbrook P, Tzika AA. Yoga and mindfulness as therapeutic interventions for stroke rehabilitation: A systematic review. Evid Based Complement Alternat Med. 2013; 2013: 357108. doi:10.1155/2013/357108.

[2] Maceira-Elvira P, Popa T, Schmid AC, Hummel FC. Wearable technology in stroke rehabilitation: towards improved diagnosis and treatment of upper-limb motor impairment. J Neuroeng Rehabil. 2019; 16(1):142. doi:10.1186/s12984-019-0612-y.

[3] Xiao-xian G, Bai-ya F, Yan-yang M. Effectiveness of neuromuscular electrical stimulation for wrist rehabilitation after acute ischemic stroke. Medicine (Baltimore) 2018; 97(38): e12299. doi: 10.1097/MD.0000000000012299.

[4] Alessandro L, Olmos LE, Bonamico L, et al. Rehabilitación multidisciplinaria para pacientes adultos con accidente cerebrovascular [Multidisciplinary rehabilitation for adult patients with stroke]. Medicina (B Aires). 2020; 80(1):54-68.

[5] Feng W, Belagaje SR. Recent advances in stroke recovery and rehabilitation. Semin Neurol. 2013; 33(5):498-506.

[6] Draaisma LR, Wessel MJ, Hummel FC. Non-invasive brain stimulation to enhance cognitive rehabilitation after stroke. Neurosci Lett. 2020; 719:133678. doi:10.1016/j.neulet.2018.06.047

[7] Jongbloed L. Prediction of function after stroke: A critical review. Stroke 1986; 17(4): 765-776.

[8] Brenner L. Effects of passive exercise training in hemiplegic stroke patients: A mini-review. Sports Med Rehabil J 2018; 3(3):Article 1036.

[9] Eng JJ. Strength training in individuals with stroke. Physiother Can. 2004;56(4):189-201. doi:10.2310/6640.2004.00025

[10] Hosseini ZS, Peyrovi H, Gohari M. The Effect of early passive range of motion exercise on motor function of people with stroke: A randomized controlled trial. J Caring Sci. 2019; 8(1):39-44. doi:10.15171/jcs.2019.006

[11] Kakuda W. Future directions of stroke rehabilitation. Rinsho Shinkeigaku. 2020; 60(3):181-186. doi:10.5692/clinicalneurol.cn-001399.

[12] Thomas LH, French B, Coupe J, McMahon N, Connell L, Harrison J, Sutton CJ, Tishkovskaya S, Watkins CL. Repetitive task training for improving functional ability after stroke: A major update of a cochrane review. Stroke. 2017; 48:e102–e103

[13] Kwakkel G, Veerbeek JM, van Wegen EE, Wolf SL. Constraint-induced movement therapy after stroke. Lancet Neurol. 2015; 14(2):224-234. doi:10.1016/S1474-4422(14)70160-7.

[14] Smith MA, Tomita MR. Combined effects of telehealth and modified constraint-induced movement therapy for individuals with chronic hemiparesis. Int J Telerehabilitation 2020; 12(1): 51-62.

[15] Thieme H, Morkisch N, Mehrholz J, Pohl M, Behrens J, Borgetto B, Dohle C. Mirror therapy for improving motor function after stroke. Cochrane Database of Systematic Reviews 2018, Issue 7. Art. No.: CD008449. DOI: 10.1002/14651858.CD008449.pub3.

[16] Gandhi DB, Sterba A, Khatter H, Pandian JD. Mirror therapy in stroke rehabilitation: Current perspectives. Ther Clin Risk Manag. 2020; 16:75-85. doi:10.2147/TCRM.S206883

[17] Hara T, Momosaki R, Niimi M, Yamada N, Hara H, Abo M. Botulinum toxin therapy combined with rehabilitation for stroke: A systematic review of effect on motor function. Toxins (Basel). 2019; 11(12):707. doi:10.3390/toxins11120707.

[18] Ozcakir S, Sivrioglu K. Botulinum toxin in poststroke spasticity. Clin Med Res. 2007; 5(2):132-138. doi:10.3121/cmr.2007.716.

[19] Forster A, Young J. Incidence and consequences of falls due to stroke: a systematic inquiry. BMJ. 1995; 311(6997): 83-86. doi:10.1136/bmj.311.6997.83.

[20] Rossano C, Terrier P. Visually-guided gait training in paretic patients during the first rehabilitation phase: study protocol for a randomized controlled trial. Trials. 2016 Oct 27; 17(1):523. doi: 10.1186/s13063-016-1630-8.

[21] Selves C, Stoquart G, Lejeune T. Gait rehabilitation after stroke: review of the evidence of predictors, clinical outcomes and timing for interventions. Acta Neurol Belg. 2020;120(4):783-790. doi:10.1007/s13760-020-01320-7

[22] Clark WE, Sivan M, O'Connor RJ. Evaluating the use of robotic and virtual reality rehabilitation technologies to improve function in stroke survivors: A narrative review. J Rehabil Assist Technol Eng. 2019;6:2055668319863557. doi:10.1177/2055668319863557.

[23] Wikipedia. Functional electrical stimulation. https://en.wikipedia.org/wiki/Functional_electrical_stimulation. Last accessed on 17 Nov 2020.

[24] Johnson M. Transcutaneous electrical nerve stimulation: mechanisms: Clinical application and evidence. Rev Pain. 2007; 1(1):7-11. doi:10.1177/204946370700100103

[25] Ito A, Kubo N, Liang N, Aoyama T, Kuroki H. regenerative rehabilitation for stroke recovery by inducing synergistic effects of cell therapy and neurorehabilitation on motor function: A narrative review of pre-clinical studies. Int J Mol Sci. 2020; 21(9):3135. doi:10.3390/ijms21093135

[26] Chang YC, Shyu WC, Lin SZ, Li H. Regenerative therapy for stroke. *Cell* Transplantation 2007; *16*(2), 171-181.

[27] Okazaki H, Beppu H, Mizutani K, Okamoto S, Sonoda S. Changes in serum growth factors in stroke rehabilitation patients and their relation to hemiparesis improvement. J Stroke Cerebrovasc Dis. 2014; 23(6):1703-1708. doi:10.1016/j.jstrokecerebrovasdis.2014.01.015

[28] Larpthaveesarp A, Ferriero DM, Gonzalez FF. Growth factors for the treatment of ischemic brain injury (growth factor treatment). Brain Sci. 2015; 5(2):165-177. doi:10.3390/brainsci5020165

[29] Szelenberger R, Kostka J, Saluk-Bijak J, Miller E. Pharmacological interventions and rehabilitation approach for enhancing brain self-repair and stroke recovery. *Curr Neuropharmacol*. 2020; 18(1):51-64. doi: 10.2174/1570159X17666190726104139.

[30] Cicerone KD, Goldin Y, Ganci K, Rosenbaum A, Wethe JV, Langenbahn DM, et al. Evidence-based cognitive rehabilitation: Systematic review of the literature from 2009 through 2014. Arch Phys Med Rehabil. 2019; 100(8):1515-1533. doi: 10.1016/j.apmr.2019.02.011.

[31] Torrisi M, Maresca G, De Cola MC, et al. Using telerehabilitation to improve cognitive function in post-stroke survivors: is this the time for the continuity of care? Int J Rehabil Res. 2019; 42(4):344-351. doi:10.1097/MRR.0000000000000369.

[32] Jelinek L, Van Quaquebeke N, Moritz S. Cognitive and metacognitive mechanisms of change in metacognitive training for depression. Sci Rep. 2017; 7(1):3449. https://doi.org/10.1038/s41598-017-03626-8.

[33] Barrett AM, Muzaffar T. Spatial cognitive rehabilitation and motor recovery after stroke. Curr Opin Neurol. 2014; 27(6):653-658.

[34] Webster BR, Celnik PA, Cohen LG. Noninvasive brain stimulation in stroke rehabilitation. NeuroRx. 2006; 3(4):474-81. doi: 10.1016/j.nurx.2006.07.008.

[35] Ovadia-Caro S, Khalil AA, Sehm B, Villringer A, Nikulin VV, Nazarova M. Predicting the response to non-invasive brain stimulation in stroke. Frontiers in Neurology 2019; 10:302. https://doi.org/10.3389/fneur.2019.00302.

[36] Wikipedia. Telerehabilitation. https://en.wikipedia.org/wiki/Telerehabilitation. Last accessed on 17 Nov 2020.

[37] Marinho DA, Neiva HP, Morais JE. The Use of Wearable Sensors in Human Movement Analysis in Non-Swimming Aquatic Activities: A Systematic Review. Int J Environ Res Public Health. 2019; 16(24):5067. doi: 10.3390/ijerph16245067.

[38] Rast FM, Labruyère R. Systematic review on the application of wearable inertial sensors to quantify everyday life motor activity in people with mobility impairments. J Neuroeng Rehabil. 2020; 17(1):148. doi: 10.1186/s12984-020-00779-y.

[39] Brennan L, Dorronzoro Zubiete E, Caulfield B. Feedback Design in Targeted Exercise Digital Biofeedback Systems for Home Rehabilitation: A Scoping Review. Sensors (Basel). 2019; 20(1):181. doi: 10.3390/s20010181

[40] Nan W, Dias APB, Rosa AC. Neurofeedback training for cognitive and motor function rehabilitation in chronic stroke: Two case reports. Front Neurol. 2019; 10:800. doi:10.3389/fneur.2019.00800

[41] Wang T, Mantini D, Gillebert CR. The potential of real-time fMRI neurofeedback for stroke rehabilitation: A systematic review. Cortex. 2018; 107:148-165. doi:10.1016/j.cortex.2017.09.006

[42] Sanchetee P, Jain A, Agarwal H. Preksha meditation and mental health in elderly. J Ind Acad Geriat 2017; 13(7): 131-138.

[43] Telles S, Naveen KV. Yoga for rehabilitation: an overview. Indian J Med Sci 1997; 51:123-7.

[44] Dein S. Religion, spirituality and neurorehabilitation. NeuroRehabilitation 2020; 46(1):1-2. doi:10.3233/NRE-200001

[45] Wikipedia. https://en.wikipedia.org/wiki/Spirituality. Accessed on 8 Sep 2020.

[46] Bastille JV, Gill-Body KM. A Yoga-based exercise program for people with chronic poststroke hemiparesis. Physical Therapy 2004; 84:33-48.

[47] Singh PS, Singh A, Mishra JPN. Management of hemiplegia through Preksha meditation. Int J Yoga Allied Sci 2014; 3:143-149.

[48] Pucciarelli G, Vellone E, Bolgeo T, Simeone S, Alvaro R, Lee CS, Lyon KS. Role of spirituality on the association between depression and quality of life in stroke survivor-care partner dyads. Circ Cardiovasc Qual Outcomes. 2020; 13(6):e006129.

[49] Immink MA, Hillier S, Petkov J. Randomized controlled trial of yoga for chronic poststroke hemiparesis:

motor function, mental health, and quality of life outcomes. Topics Stroke Rehabilitation 2014; 21(3), 256-271.

[50] Lynton H, Kligler B, Shiflett S. Yoga in stroke rehabilitation: a systematic review and results of a pilot study. Top Stroke Rehabil. 2007; 14(4):1-8. doi: 10.1310/tsr1404-1.

[51] Silveira K, Smart CM. Cognitive, physical, and psychological benefits of yoga for acquired brain injuries: A systematic review of recent findings. Neuropsychol Rehabil. 2020; 30(7):1388-1407. doi:10.1080/09602011.2019.1583114.

[52] Gothe NP, Khan I, Hayes J, Erlenbach E, Damoiseauxb JS. Yoga effects on brain health: A systematic review of the current literature. Brain Plast. 2019; 5(1): 105-122. doi: 10.3233/BPL-190084

[53] Venditti S, Verdone L, Reale A, Vetriani V, Caserta M, Zampieri M. Molecules of silence: effects of meditation on gene expression and epigenetics. Front Psychol. 2020; 11:1767. doi:10.3389/fpsyg.2020.01767

Chapter 2

Ischemic Stroke in Young Adults: Practical Diagnosis Guide

Diana Mihai, Florentina Cristina Plesa, Any Docu Axelerad, Alice Munteanu, Minerva Claudia Ghinescu and Carmen Adella Sirbu

Abstract

With its increasing incidence in younger population and as a leading cause of disability, ischemic stroke represents a real public health problem. This chapter aims to evaluate the most common risk factors and causes for ischemic stroke in the young. Though some are identical to those found in older patients, most of them are specific to this population segment. Furthermore, another objective is to provide some guidance in approaching the case based on some important clinical clues. Due to the lack of universal management guidelines, it is up to the physician to judge the particularities of each case and to carry out the variety of investigations necessary for determining the cause.

Keywords: ischemic stroke, young adults, risk factors, etiology, diagnosis guide

1. Introduction

Contrary to the general opinion that it is a disease of the elderly, ischemic stroke is a condition that can occur at any age. Of course, its incidence increases with age, but it has been observed to increasingly affect young people. This tendency can have multiple consequences. Since it targets the young working population, economic and social burden are known to appear.

Although some of the causes or risk factors of ischemic stroke are common for both young and elderly patients, they do not overlap. In young people, the causes can be multiple: heart, vascular, or genetic disorders that require further, sometimes complex investigations. In addition, most cryptogenic strokes appear in this age category. The classic cardiovascular risk factors, which are in present much more prevalent at much younger ages, should also be taken into account.

This chapter aims to illustrate the most frequent causes of ischemic stroke in young people and its associated risk factors and to provide some guidance regarding further investigations necessary for determining the cause.

2. Ischemic stroke in young adults

2.1 Epidemiology

Stroke represents a common cause of morbidity and mortality worldwide. It has been estimated that more than 11 million patients are diagnosed with ischemic stroke each year [1]. The incidence of stroke varies by geographical area and also by sex, age, and race. Although stroke has been previously considered a disease that is mostly affecting the older population, recent publications show that between 10 and 15% of the total number of strokes occur in younger patients [2]. This means that each year, approximately 2 million adolescents and young adults across the world suffer from an ischemic stroke [3]. Furthermore, recent epidemiological studies have shown that since the 1980s, the incidence of ischemic stroke in the young population has increased, while its incidence in the elderly group has declined. This result raises a few concerns regarding its socioeconomic impact. It occurs in young people with long-life spans ahead, during their most productive years, and causes major long-term disability, with great health-care costs [4]. Some possible explanations for this trend are: improved population awareness regarding stroke symptoms, improved diagnosis performance using advanced neuroimaging techniques, or an increment in the prevalence of the known risk factors (type 2 diabetes, obesity, lack of physical activity, and recreational drug use).

An important question is how is this "young stroke" group defined? Which are its cut-off limits? The majority of authors are using the age of 45 as the group's upper limit [5]. Others favor the age of 49 [2]. This age limit has been arbitrarily drawn based on the major differences in etiologies and risk factors between these two age groups [1].

It has been found that the incidence rate of stroke grows with age, being at its highest in the 45–49 age interval and at its lowest in the group of patients younger than 35 [4].

Incidence rates vary also from a geographical perspective. Developing countries report a higher incidence rate than industrialized ones [1]. Asian countries such as Japan and Taiwan also report higher rates [5]. The "young stroke" incidence is also higher among American blacks and Hispanics. In addition, it has been stated that the hospital stay was longer and mortality higher in black population versus Caucasian [1].

Looking at sex differences, the incidence appears to be higher in men than in women, though some studies have shown that before the age of 30 the incidence of "young stroke" is higher in women [5]. Men have exhibited a higher mortality rate and risk for reoccurring vascular events [1].

2.2 Pathophysiology of ischemic stroke

An ischemic stroke occurs due to a decreased blood flow in a certain area in the brain. This can be the consequences of obstruction of one of the blood vessels that irrigates the brain, or it can occur due to low systemic blood pressure. The most common causes of blood vessel obstruction are thrombosis and embolization. Thrombosis usually develops on atherosclerotic plaques. Atherosclerotic plaques tend to form in larger arteries and are responsible for narrowing the vascular lumen. The process can even lead to the complete occlusion of the blood vessel. The blood clot can embolize distally, causing an ischemic stroke. Though rarely, in situ thrombosis can also occur due to an underlying hematological abnormality (leukemia and polycythemia). Other causes of arterial obstruction are arteritis, arterial dissection, and arteriolosclerosis. Distal embolization is another common mechanism. Most commonly, the source is cardiac. When the source of emboli is in the venous system of the members, the correct term is paradoxical embolization.

When discussing the pathophysiology of ischemic stroke, we most often refer to arterial stroke [6]. Cerebral blood flow (CBF) represents the ratio of cerebral blood volume (CBV) to mean transit time (MTT). There is a directly proportional relationship between CBF reduction and the size of the stroke. Narrowing the vessel caliber, MTT increases and CBF decreases. To minimize the reduction in blood flow, autoregulation mechanisms start to intervene. Distally to the site of occlusion or stenosis, vasodilation appears, and in addition, the oxygen extraction rate increases. These initial measures help maintain normal perfusion. CBF of 50 ml/100 g brain tissue/min represents the adequate cerebral blood supply. In the ischemic penumbra, FSC is somewhere between 10 and 30 ml/100 g brain tissue/min. The nerve cells in this area can be saved in the first hours after symptoms onset by methods of recanalization of the affected vessel. When FSC drops below 10 ml/100 g of brain tissue, necrosis occurs. The nerve cells in the necrotized area can, at this point, no longer be recovered. ATP depletion, high extracellular K levels, high intracellular Ca levels, cellular acidosis, phospholipases activation, intracellular enzymes, and structural protein alteration eventually lead to cytotoxic edema and cell death. Neural losses are irreversible and begin in the first 4–8 minutes after the onset of ischemia, in the absence of collateral circulation to supplement the cerebral blood flow. In every minute of ischemia, 1.9 million neurons, 14 million synapses, and 12 km of myelin fibers are lost [7].

However, a small fraction of ischemic strokes is caused by venous blood flow abnormalities. Intracranial venous occlusion can cause hemorrhages and compressions and can lead to ischemia [6].

2.3 Risk factors

Conventional cardiovascular risk factors, for instance, hypertension, diabetes, and dyslipidemia, are considered important risk factors for all adults. Their prevalence among the young has been increasing over the last 10 years. Studies show that the most common risk factors found among young stroke patients are: smoking (56%), physical inactivity (48%), hypertension (47%), and dyslipidemia (35%) [2, 4]. On the other hand, among the elderly, the most prevalent ones are hypertension, diabetes, and cardiac diseases such as atrial fibrillation [8]. The tendency toward obesity, the lack of physical activity, the rising number of smokers, and heavy episodic alcohol consumption among teenagers and young adults, which have all been linked to a higher ischemic stroke incidence, are, indeed, worrisome [1].

An interesting observation is that young patients with no vascular risk factors have lower mortality associated with the stroke and fewer recurrences. This means that the number of vascular risk factors can be regarded as an important prognostic factor to determine clinical outcome [8].

Drug use is another important risk factor. It is believed that roughly 5% of the population aged 15–64 use illicit or recreational drugs at least once a year. Such substances associated with ischemic stroke are cocaine, amphetamine, cannabis, and opioids. The negative effects of these substances can be explained either through their direct effects on the cardiovascular system or through complications linked to their administration pathway (embolism or endocarditis related to intravenous administration). The negative effects on cardiovascular system include cardiomyopathies, cardiac arrhythmias, orthostatic hypotension, vasoconstriction, platelet aggregation, accelerated atherosclerosis, and vasculitis. Though previously thought harmless, cannabis consumption can possibly lead to reversible cerebral vasoconstriction syndrome and intimal hyperplasia [3, 8].

Pregnancy and the puerperium are also associated with an elevated risk for ischemic events. Although considered a somewhat scarce occurrence, ischemic strokes associated with pregnancy carry higher mortality rates. The risk is at its highest from the third trimester until 6 weeks postpartum [9]. In countries like India and Mexico, pregnancy-related stroke is not that uncommon and is caused by dural sinus thrombosis [10]. Causes of ischemic stroke in this category of patients are peripartum cardiomyopathy, hypercoagulability associated with pregnancy, postpartum cerebral angiopathy (reversible cerebral vasoconstriction syndrome), amniotic fluid embolism, or trophoblastic embolism due to choriocarcinoma [9]. Ischemic stroke during pregnancy is also linked to other pregnancy-related complications, as the mechanisms appear to be similar [3]. Special attention should be given to peripartum cerebral venous thrombosis. Risk factors are anemia, first time carrying a pregnancy, and lack of medical care during pregnancy. Frequent signs and symptoms at presentation for patients with this condition are headache, altered consciousness, and motor deficit. Papilledema is observed in up to 80% of patients. Treatment includes anticoagulation, and sometimes, anticonvulsant therapy is also necessary. Prognosis is usually favorable [11].

Contraceptive use raises the risk of ischemic stroke, even more so if associated with smoking or migraines with aura. The risk is tightly linked to the estrogen content in the pill. Progesterone contraceptives do not pose any threat [5, 8].

Migraine with aura appears to be linked to ischemic stroke, especially if tied with other risk factors such as smoking and use of oral estrogen contraceptives. The association is, though, quite controversial [2, 3]. The mechanism is still not known. Its involvement as a risk factor is more evident in young women [5].

Malignancy, along with chemotherapy and radiotherapy, can increase the risk of ischemic stroke, through various mechanisms: direct vessel compression, tumor embolism, nonbacterial thrombotic endocarditis, hypercoagulability, and accelerated atherosclerosis. Current guidelines offer no information regarding cancer screening in young patients presenting for stroke [3].

2.4 Etiology

2.4.1 Cardiac causes

Cardiac embolism is responsible for almost 30% of ischemic strokes in young adults [8]. The most frequent causes of cardiac embolism are presented in **Table 1**.

Although regarded as a frequent risk factor in the elderly, atrial fibrillation is not as prevalent in the young [2]. Due to its paroxysmal occurrence, it is also relatively difficult to diagnose, and it requires continuous monitoring, which is not always justified in younger patients with no cardiac pathology. Other electrocardiographic abnormalities regarding the P-wave have also been associated with higher risk for ischemic stroke [3, 8]. Due to rheumatic heart disease, mitral valve disease should be considered as a potential cause of ischemic stroke in the young. Its prevalence is higher in less industrialized geographic areas [5].

Cardiomyopathies, though rare, should also be considered. Dilated cardiomyopathy is linked to alcohol consumption and occurs at younger age. Chagas disease is more frequent in South America [5]. HIV-associated cardiomyopathy has also been cited as a possible etiology [12]. Peripartum cardiomyopathy is frequent in sub-Saharan Africa. In this case, an echocardiography can help identify the source of emboli [3]. An echocardiography can also identify a cardiac tumor as a source of emboli, such as an atrial myxoma or a papillary fibroelastoma. Atrial myxoma is the most common type of cardiac tumor. It is usually asymptomatic and only discovered after an ischemic stroke. Ischemic stroke can also be a complication of infectious or thrombotic nonbacterial endocarditis. Infectious endocarditis should be suspected particularly if the patient is an intravenous drug user. Thrombosis due to acute myocardial infarction or congestive heart failure is not common causes in young-related ischemic stroke [13]. Patent foramen ovale is a frequent congenital anomaly, found in over 20% of the population. Its prevalence in stroke patients

Cardioembolic cause	
Lower prevalence	**Higher prevalence**
Atrial fibrillation	Congenital cardiac anomalies • Patent foramen ovale • Atrial septal aneurysms
Nonrheumatic valvular disease	Cardiomyopathies
Acute myocardial infarction	Rheumatic valvular disease
Cardiac tumors	Endocarditis

Table 1.
Cardioembolic causes of stroke in the young.

younger than 50 years old is even higher, up to 50%, but its direct role as a causative agent is still debated [8]. Patent foramen ovale is not solely responsible for such consequences, and it also requires other contributing factors such as the simultaneous presence of an atrial septal aneurysm, at rest right to left shunt, larger shunt. Furthermore, additional risk factors for venous thrombosis should be present: prolonged immobilization, long distance travel, varicose veins, trauma, or prothrombotic conditions [4].

To determine whether PFO was the main mechanism in patients with stroke, it is useful to calculate the Risk of Paradoxical Embolism (RoPE) score [14].

The RoPE score (**Table 2**) ranges between 0 and 10 points. A higher score indicates a strong possibility that PFO is the causative agent, while a lower score suggests that PFO could only be an incidental find (**Figure 1**) [4]. RoPE score can also predict the risk of recurrence. A patient with a high RoPE score is a young patient with very few to almost no cardiovascular risk factor and, as a consequence, a very low short-term recurrence risk [3].

2.4.2 Nonatherosclerotic, noninflammatory angiopathies

Cervicocephalic arterial dissection is the origin of ischemic stroke in young patients in 20% of the cases. It affects men in a larger proportion than women (52–69%) [15]. It refers to the intramural hemorrhage of the extracranial arterial segments. The vertebral artery and the internal carotid artery are affected in 90% of the cases [16]. Their cervical extracranial segments are most susceptible to dissection due to their mobility and close proximity to adjacent bone structures such as the transverse processes of the cervical vertebrae. The site of dissection is different than the segment usually affected by the process of atherosclerosis. While atherosclerosis usually develops at the origin of the internal carotid artery, the arterial segments prone to dissection are the distal cervical segments of the internal carotid artery. The vertebral artery, more mobile and prone to injury, is also most affected at its distal extracranial segment, the V3 segment [15, 17].

As a result of a tear in the intimal layer of the vessel, an intramural hematoma will appear. The blood then further extends superiorly along the longitudinal axis of the blood vessel. The hematoma develops between the layers of the media, but if it is situated between the intimal layer and media, the dissection is called subintimal. This type of dissections will most likely narrow the arterial lumen and cause stenosis or even full occlusion of the artery. However, if the blood enters between the tunica media and the adventitia, a dissection aneurysm will occur. This type of dissection is called subadventitial. In this type of dissection, the arterial lumen is not narrowed, and it actually appears widened and can compress adjacent

Patient information	Points
Cortical stroke	1
No hypertension	1
No diabetes	1
No previous stroke or TIA	1
Nonsmoker	1
AGE	
18–29	5
30–39	4
40–49	3
50–59	2
60–69	1
>70	0
Total	

Table 2.
RoPE score [14].

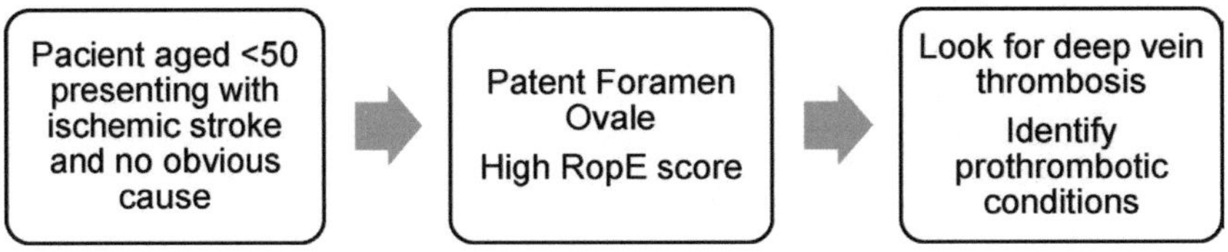

Figure 1.
Pathway to determining etiology of ischemic stroke in patients with PFO.

structures such as sympathetic nerves or the hypoglossal cranial nerve. A blood clot typically forms at the segment of artery affected. The thrombus is not firmly attached to the intimal layer and can easily embolize distally [15, 16, 18]. Dissection of the carotid or vertebral arteries can be accompanied by several signs or symptoms. Headache and neck pain are common. Ipsilateral Claude Bernard Horner Syndrome can occur due to compression of the hematoma on the adjacent sympathetic nerve fibers. Ipsilateral cranial nerve palsies can also be present. These signs can precede the ischemic event with hours or even days in some cases [19].

Predisposing factors to cervicocephalic arterial dissection are: hypertension, recent infection, and migraine. Surprisingly, risk factors for atherosclerosis such as obesity and dyslipidemia are negatively correlated with cervical arteries dissection [19].

A cervicocephalic arterial dissection can appear spontaneously (in 60% of the cases) or after a recent traumatic event [15]. The traumatic events possibly responsible and other risk factors are illustrated in **Table 3**.

Furthermore, arterial dissection can occur on a normally structured blood vessel or on a vessel affected by an underlying arteriopathy (**Table 3**).

An ultrasound examination can suggest the presence of arterial dissections, but the diagnosis is made through angio-magnetic resonance imaging and angio-computer tomography.

Angiography, though an invasive procedure, is the most accurate and precise diagnostic tool.

Underlying nonatherosclerotic, noninflammatory arteriopathies	
Fibromuscular dysplasia	
Moyamoya disease	
Type 4 Ehlers-Danlos syndrome	
Osteogenesis imperfecta type 1	
Pseudoxanthoma elasticum	
Autosomal dominant polycystic kidney disease	
α1-antitrypsin deficiency	
Mechanical trigger factors for cervicocephalic arterial dissection	
Major traumatic events	Cervical spine fracture
	Direct trauma to the anterior neck (punch, strangling)
	Penetrating lesion of the anterior neck
	Sudden and severe rotations of the neck
Minor traumatic events	Sports activities (skiing, tennis, and yoga)
	Forceful coughing
	Vomiting
	Nose blowing
	Sexual activity
	Abnormal, sustained head position
	Prolonged head turning
Iatrogenic cause	Chiropractic manipulation of the neck
	Resuscitation
	Anesthesia

Table 3.
Underlying nonatherosclerotic, noninflammatory arteriopathies and mechanical trigger factors for cervicocephalic arterial dissection.

2.4.3 Inflammatory diseases

The term vasculitis groups a series of diseases characterized by inflammation of blood vessel walls. Inflammation of blood vessels, possibly accompanied by varying degrees of necrosis, can lead to stenosis, vessel occlusion, or aneurysmal dilation. Both arteries and veins can be affected, regardless of their size. Vasculitis that affects the central nervous system can be either primary or secondary to a systemic disorder [19].

Primary angiitis of the central nervous system (PACNS) usually affects small vessels (precapillary arterioles). The lesions are multifocal, which makes it difficult to diagnose. A normal biopsy does not rule out PACNS. It can affect both brain and spinal cord, but no other organs are affected. Its evolution is heterogenic, but it usually presents in a recurrent remitting fashion. Sometimes, it can be rapidly progressive, leading to exitus in a matter of days [20]. The cause of PACNS is not known, but studies show that it is usually associated with other diseases such as Hodgkin lymphoma, leukemia, primary intracerebral lymphoma, HIV infection, and Varicella Zoster virus infection. Most frequently, the clinical picture includes headache and altered cognition, sometimes seizures. Systemic symptoms and signs such as fever, fatigue, weakness, loss of appetite, and weight loss are very rarely seen. Blood inflammatory markers such as C-reactive protein and erythrocyte sedimentation rate (ESR) are usually normal or slightly elevated. So is blood cell count. The cerebrospinal fluid analysis shows signs of inflammation.

Many systemic vasculitides can affect the central nervous system. Some of the most common are briefly presented in **Table 4**. Other causes of noninfectious angiitis include drug use, radiotherapy, and neoplasia [20].

When the central nervous system is affected, the clinical picture typically includes headaches. Other signs and symptoms that may be suggestive are fever, weight loss, dermatological findings (rash and livedo reticularis), articular lesions, and kidney disease. The inflammation markers such as C-reactive protein and ESR are usually elevated. Other frequent findings in blood tests are anemia, thrombocytopenia, and low complement levels. Cerebrospinal fluid also shows increased level of proteins and inflammatory cells [19].

In a young patient presenting with ischemic stroke with accompanying suggestive symptoms, a systemic angiitis should be suspected. Determining ANCAs and dsDNA antibodies can, in this particular case, be of an important value for determining an underlying condition causing the stroke (**Figure 2**) [21].

2.4.4 Infectious diseases

Some infectious diseases are linked through various mechanisms with ischemic stroke. Some infectious agents tied to secondary vasculitis are presented in **Table 5**. Infections involved in the pathogenesis can be either viral, bacterial, parasitic, or fungal [22].

HIV infections can predispose to stroke through various mechanisms. One pathogenic pathway is large vessel HIV arteriopathy. The arteriopathy may be due to the direct pathogenic effect of the virus. As a consequence of the vasculopathy, large, hemispheric infarctions can appear. Another possible pathogenic pathway is through opportunistic infections of the central nervous system, which can occur as HIV is responsible for an immunosuppressive state. Such opportunistic infections are tuberculosis, Varicella-Zoster virus infection, toxoplasmosis, and syphilis [20].

Tuberculous meningitis is a severe condition with a high mortality rate. Up to 45% of patients diagnosed with tuberculous meningitis develop a stroke, sometimes even multiple strokes [20, 22].

Systemic angiitis affecting the central nervous system	
Large-vessel angiitis	Takayasu's disease
Medium-vessel angiitis	Polyarteritis nodosa
	Kawasaki disease
Small-vessel angiitis ANCA +	Eosinophilic granulomatosis with polyangiitis (Churg-Strauss syndrome)
	Granulomatosis with polyangiitis (Wegener granulomatosis)
	Microscopic polyangiitis
Angiitis associated with connective tissue disease	Systemic lupus erythematosus
	Rheumatoid arthritis
	Behçet disease

Table 4.
Systemic angiitis that affects the central nervous system.

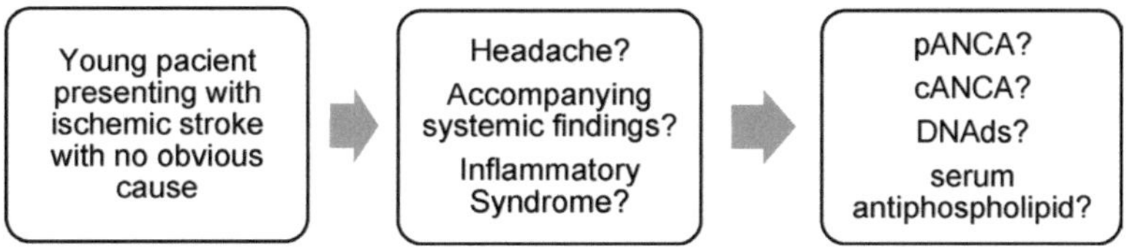

Figure 2.
Pathway to determine etiology in young patients with ischemic stroke.

Infectious agents linked to secondary vasculitis	
Viral infections	HIV (AIDS) Hepatitis B and C Varicella-Zoster virus infection Cytomegalovirus infection
Bacterial infections	Tuberculosis Lyme neuroborreliosis Bacterial meningitis Syphilis Mycoplasma pneumoniae infection Brucellosis
Parasitic infections	Cysticercosis Chagas disease Trypanosoma cruzi infection Leptospirosis Malaria
Fungal infections	Cryptococcus infection Aspergillus infection

Table 5.
Infectious agents linked to secondary vasculitis [2, 20].

Among parasitic infections, Chagas disease and cysticercosis are most commonly involved. Up to 10% of the patients with neurocysticercosis develop strokes (ischemic strokes occur more frequently) [20, 22].

Fungal infections most commonly affect patients who suffer from immunosuppression. Ischemic strokes represent an unfortunate complication. Cryptococcus infections and aspergillosis are linked to HIV infection [20].

In the present context of Covid-19 pandemic, it is important to emphasize the link between the infection and a prothrombotic status. Thrombotic complications represent a frequent find in patients infected. For this reason, the risk of ischemic strokes should also be taken into consideration [23].

2.4.5 Hematological diseases

A large number of hematological diseases predispose to stroke. The mechanisms behind this predisposition are increased blood viscosity, which in return decreases blood flow and hypercoagulability. Even though, a single factor cannot by itself be the only cause for the ischemic stroke, a combination of such predisposing factors can have such unwanted consequences. Some conditions that lead to an increase in blood viscosity are leukemia, intravascular lymphoma, sickle cell anemia, erythrocytosis, polycythemia vera, Waldenström's macroglobulinemia, paraproteinemia, and spherocytosis. Even though coagulopathies are mostly associated with venous thrombosis, recent studies show that deficiency in certain factors involved in blood clotting such as Protein C, Protein S, antithrombin, and Factor V Leiden mutation increases the risk of arterial thrombosis [19].

Factor V Leiden mutation is a single point mutation that leads to protein C activity resistance. The result is generation of high levels of thrombin, which in turn raises the risk for thromboembolic events. Heterozygosity or homozygosity for this mutation is usually associated with other hereditary coagulation abnormalities [24].

Prothrombin gene mutation is another frequent hereditary disease that interferes with normal blood coagulation. Patients with prothrombin gene mutation have higher than normal levels of prothrombin, which predisposes to thrombosis. This condition is associated with cerebral venous thrombosis, especially when there is a second risk factor involved, like the use of oral contraceptives [24].

Protein C and Protein S are proteins that inhibit the coagulation cascade. Their deficiency predisposes to blood coagulation and can be genetic, or, in some cases, acquired. Conditions associated with Protein C and Protein S deficiency are contraceptives use, pregnancy, severe infections, liver diseases, disseminated intravascular coagulation, and certain medications such as methotrexate and cyclophosphamide [24].

Antithrombin III (ATIII) deficiency is a genetic disease inherited in an autosomal-dominant pattern. Its prevalence in the population is 0.2%. Its role is to inhibit the generation of thrombin. Antithrombin deficiency can also be acquired: severe infections, cirrhosis, disseminated intravascular coagulation, and nephrotic syndrome [24].

None of the conditions described above (Factor V Leiden mutation, prothrombin gene mutation, Protein C and S deficiency, and ATIII deficiency) can cause, by themselves, without additional risk factors, in situ arterial thrombosis. On the other hand, Antiphospholipid Antibody Syndrome is known to cause venous, as well as arterial thrombosis. Ischemic stroke is a recognized complication of this syndrome [24].

2.4.6 Genetic diseases

Family history of stroke at a young age should be suggestive for a genetic cause. Many genetic abnormalities have been linked to the possibility of ischemic stroke. However, stroke represents the main manifestation in only a few genetic diseases.

Periventricular lesions with predominant temporal pole involvement may suggest an autosomal dominant arteriopathy with subcortical infarcts and leukoencephalopathy CADASIL, with autosomal dominant transmission. Although rare, it is an undiagnosed affliction, so its prevalence may be underestimated. The condition is characterized by a mutation in the NOTCH3 gene located on chromosome 19. The NOTCH3 gene is expressed almost exclusively in smooth muscle fibers and encodes a receptor located at the cell surface. NOTCH3 gene mutation leads to smooth muscle degeneration. The condition starts manifesting between the age of 30 and 60. Patients present with recurrent ischemic strokes, migraine with aura, mood swings, and progressive cognitive impairment. Severe leukoaraiosis is seen on imagining. Temporal lobes are typically involved [19, 25].

Cerebral autosomal recessive arteriopathy with subcortical infarcts and leukoencephalopathy (CARASIL) is a much rare disease than CADASIL and affects almost exclusively the Japanese population. It is characterized by a mutation in HTRA1 gene, which encodes HtrA serine peptidase/protease 1 (HTRA1). The clinical picture includes alopecia occurring at young age, low back pain, progressive cognitive impairment, and lacunar strokes [19, 26].

CARASAL is another vascular leukoencephalopathy with R325C mutation in CTSA gene [27].

In other genetic diseases, such as Fabry disease or homocystinuria, though not considered a representative feature, ischemic stroke is strongly linked. Fabry disease has X-linked transmission. It is characterized by a reduced activity of the α-galactosidase enzyme, an enzyme involved in lipid metabolism. As a result, lysosomal lipid accumulation occurs in endothelial cells and smooth muscle fibers of blood vessels. This process can have many unwanted consequences, including ischemic stroke. The diagnosis is made by dosing the enzyme value in patient's blood.

Homocystinuria is a genetic disease transmitted in an autosomal recessive pattern and characterized by high levels of homocysteine in blood and urine. The cause is a deficit in an enzyme called cystathionine β-synthase. The clinical picture includes Marfanoid appearance, mental retardation, premature atherosclerosis, and thrombembolic events.

MELAS (mitochondrial encephalopathy, lactic acidosis, and stroke-like episodes) is caused by mutations in mitochondrial DNA. Ischemic strokes appear before the age of 40. The occipital lobes are typically affected [26].

2.4.7 Venous ischemic stroke in young

Cerebral venous thrombosis (CVT) is a rare affliction, occurring mostly in the younger population. Seventy-five percent of the patients diagnosed with CVT are young women [19]. Even though if mostly affects young women, it can occur at any age, children and newborns also being affected.

Hormones clearly play a role in the pathophysiology of the disease. Its incidence is higher during pregnancy and postpartum (especially in countries such as India and Mexico). It is also correlated with oral contraceptive use and other hormonal therapies [28].

Other risk factors for CVS are hematological diseases that cause blood hypercoagulation and other coagulopathies, infections of the central nervous system, sinus and ear infections or other infections occurring in the region of head and neck, and severe systemic infections (HIV, tuberculosis, and sepsis). Malignancy, systemic inflammatory diseases such as SLE and sarcoidosis and several inflammatory angiopathies are also linked to CVT. Other events linked to CVT are head trauma, brain surgery, and lumbar punctures [29].

The obstruction of dural venous sinuses or intracerebral veins hinders blood drainage and leads to increased pressure above the obstacle. As a result, in the affected area of the brain, edema develops. Arterioles and capillaries can break and hemorrhage appears. In addition, if the tissue pressure becomes higher than the arteriole's pressure of perfusion, ischemia installs [28].

Transverse sinuses and superior sagittal sinuses are most affected. Sometimes, multiple areas in the brain can be affected [19].

The clinical onset is typically gradual, but a sudden onset is also possible. The clinical picture includes headache, seizures, focal neurological signs, and altered consciousness. A useful sign is the presence of papilledema.

Blood tests show elevated D-dimer levels.

Neuroimaging is the most helpful tool in the diagnosis process. A CT scan can visualize parenchymal hemorrhage and tissue edema. Sometimes, the thrombus can be seen on imaging as a hyperdense lesion. MRI is an even more sensitive method, which can better characterize the abnormalities in the brain parenchyma. It can reveal recent infarction, hemorrhage, and tissue edema. These imaging techniques also help identify some predisposing factors such as sinusitis, mastoiditis, cerebral tumors, or abscesses. They are also extremely useful in the differential diagnosis process [28].

CVS is a condition that can now benefit from rapid diagnosis with IRM techniques. When rapidly identified and specific measures applied, the prognosis is favorable, the condition having a low mortality rate [19].

Anticoagulation is the therapy of choice, even if imaging also shows hemorrhage. Thrombolytic therapy has not proved to be superior to anticoagulation. It is used only when anticoagulating agents fail. Sometimes, when the etiology of thrombosis is identified, it may require specific treatment. The patient may require antibacterial or antiviral therapy, antineoplastic agents. In case of severe cases of raised intracranial pressure, decompression techniques may be performed [28].

2.4.8 Cryptogenic stroke

Despite all the diagnostic advances, up to 35% of ischemic strokes, especially in young people, have no identified cause [20].

2.5 Diagnosis

For determining the underlying cause of ischemic stroke in the young, certain clinical clues can be of great value (**Table 6**). Depending on the clinical picture, routine investigations can be then followed by additional, more specific tests (**Table** 7) [19, 20, 30].

Apart from the usual test in young patients presenting with ischemic stroke (complete blood count, blood glucose, hemoglobin a1c, lipid panel, heart enzymes CK, troponin, electrocardiogram, liver and kidney function, ESR, CRP, serum electrolytes, PT, INR, APTT, pregnancy test, urine analysis, brain imaging, and chest X-ray), specific ones will be made depending on the diagnostic suspicion (**Table** 7) [20, 30].

2.6 Differential diagnosis of ischemic stroke

There are many conditions (vascular or nonvascular) that may simulate an acute ischemic stroke. One study reveals that 14% of patients that had presented with acute neurological deficits were falsely diagnosed with ischemic stroke and received thrombolytic medication. The reevaluation proved to be, in fact, a stroke mimic. The differential diagnosis may differ depending on the age of the patient. In general, in a young patient presenting with sudden focal deficit, the following should be taken into consideration: hemorrhagic stroke, cerebral venous thrombosis, complicated migraine, seizures, acute vestibular syndrome, central nervous system tumor or abscess, multiple sclerosis, myasthenia gravis, alcohol intoxication, drug or medication toxicity, hypo or hyperglycemia, dyselectrolytemia, uremia, hyperthyroidism, hepatic encephalopathy, hypertensive encephalopathy, Wernicke encephalopathy, cardiac syncope and psychiatric disorders [10, 31, 32].

2.7 Treatment and prognosis

The clinical presentation, treatment, and clinical outcome depend on the type and cause of stroke. After the etiology of stroke is identified, management and prevention are individualized [2].

The therapy of choice remains intravenous thrombolysis with recombinant tissue plasminogen activator. Young patients tend to have fewer complications, if the therapy is administered faster and the outcome is favorable. Bleeding risk is substantially decreased. The delay between presentation and therapy initiation is usually caused by difficulties in diagnosis [33].

Clinical clue	Suspicion
Fever	Infection Connective tissue disease Vasculitis
Lymphadenopathy	Lymphoma Infection
History of asthma	Churg Strauss syndrome
History of recent head trauma	Arterial dissection In situ arterial thrombosis
Headache	Hereditary endotheliopathy, retinopathy, nephropathy, and stroke (HERNS) Cerebral autosomal dominant arteriopathy with subcortical infarcts and leukoencephalopathy (CADASIL) Reversible cerebral vasoconstriction syndrome (RCVS) Arterial dissection Vasculitis Systemic lupus erythematosum (SLE)
Acroparesthesia	Fabry disease
Erythema migrans	Lyme disease
Oral/genital ulcers	Syphilis SLE Behçet disease Herpes simplex
Angiokeratomas	Fabry disease
Erythema nodosum	Connective tissue disease Tuberculosis Poststreptococcal infections Sarcoidosis Behçet disease
Butterfly erythema	SLE
Splinter hemorrhages underneath the nail	Endocarditis
Raynaud syndrome	Connective tissue disease Neoplasia Blood hyperviscosity
Needle puncture signs	Drug use
Tattoos	HIV infection Hepatitis
Alopecia	Systemic lupus erythematosus (SLE) Temporal arteritis Cerebral autosomal recessive arteriopathy with subcortical infarcts and leukoencephalopathy (CARASIL)
Xanthelasma	Hyperlipidemia
Decreased vision	Mitochondrial disease HERNS Pseudoxanthoma elasticum
Claude Bernard Horner Syndrome	Carotid dissection
Dry eyes	Sjögren syndrome
Iritis	Behçet disease
Roth spots	Endocarditis

Table 6.
Clinical clues in ischemic stroke in the young.

Additional investigations	
Blood/urine toxicology	**Drug use**
Arterial blood gas analysis	MELAS
Rheumatoid factor Complement level dsDNA antibodies ANA antibodies Anti Ro, anti La antibodies Scl 70 antibody Anticentromere antibody Anticardiolipin antibodies Cryoglobulins Serum angiotensin-converting enzyme	Connective tissue disease/other rheumatic diseases
ANCA antibodies Fluorescein angiography	Systemic angiitis
Electrophoresis	Paraproteinemia
Hemoglobin electrophoresis	Sickle cell disease
Specific tests for syphilis, tuberculosis, herpes, HIV, Lyme, and hepatitis	Infectious disease
D-dimers	Thromboembolism
Protein S, Protein C, Factor V Leiden, antithrombin, prothrombin gene mutation	Coagulation abnormalities
Echocardiography	Patent foramen ovale Cardiomyopathy Endocarditis
Holter electrocardiogram	Atrial fibrillation
Lower extremity ultrasonography (in patients with PFO)	Deep vein thrombosis
Coombs test	Hematologic abnormalities
Bone marrow biopsy	Hematologic abnormalities
Cerebrospinal fluid examination (cellularity, glucose, proteins, oligoclonal bands, and infectious agents)	
Arterial/skin/muscle biopsy	Giant cell arteritis CADASIL CARASIL Mitochondrial disease
Brain biopsy	Primary cerebral vasculitides
α-Galactosidase enzyme level	Fabry disease
Homocysteine level	Homocystinuria
Genetic tests	CARASIL/CADASIL and others
Advanced imaging techniques	Personalized, depending on clinical suspicion

Table 7.
Specific additional investigations for young stroke etiology.

Studies show that the mortality in young stroke patients is up to four times higher in the first 20 years after the stroke than healthy people [3]. It has also been observed that cardiac insufficiency and stroke severity are important mortality predictors [2].

Because we are referring to a younger, still employed population, the socioeconomic burden cannot be neglected. We learn from studies that up to one third of patients who suffered an ischemic stroke remain unemployed even up to 8 years after the episode. This may be due to the disability or solely the consequence of depression. Depression following the stroke is a frequent find between this segment of patients, along with chronic fatigue and anxiety [3]. In addition, depression has been shown to also influence mortality [30]. Some other long-term consequences that have to be taken into consideration are chronic central pain, sexual dysfunction, cognitive impairment, and epileptic syndrome. Due to this multiple possible consequences, the patients' approach should be multidisciplinary, including a neurologist, a psychologist or a psychiatrist, and an occupational therapist [3].

Another important aspect is the risk of recurrence. Cardioembolic strokes or patients suffering from atherosclerosis affecting the large vessels are the ones most at risk for recurrence [3].

2.8 Rehabilitation after stroke

The rehabilitation process of stroke victims is extremely complex. It is not limited only to the medical part of the process, but also includes social, economic, and vocational aspects. It is important to keep in mind that the patient rehabilitation should be achieved through a multidisciplinary approach, with a team of specialists from different domains of activity: physicians, nurses, physiotherapists, speech-language therapists, social workers, and occupational therapists [34].

The methods used for rehabilitation are similar between the young and the elderly. It has been observed that younger people tend to achieve a full recovery after stroke more frequently and more rapidly and require institutionalization less frequently than older patients. The main predictors of full recovery after stroke are age and stroke severity. On the other hand, younger patients struggle more with adjustment issues, family stress, vocational issues, and depression. For this reason, rehabilitation in younger people should focus on issues regarding disease acceptance and community integration. It is of uttermost importance for these patients to be informed about their disease, about possible future consequences, including stroke recurrence. Including these patients in support groups of stroke victims of similar age would also be extremely useful [35].

The rehabilitation program can be performed in acute care hospitals, in different rehabilitation centers, or even at home. In absence of contraindications, rehabilitation should begin as early as possible. Early mobilization, when possible, is also recommended in the first 18–24 hours. The process is individualized depending on patient's disabilities and focuses on improving cognitive, motor, and speech skills. Motor rehabilitation includes different techniques to improve mobility, balance, sit-to-stand, gait, and upper limb function and limit spasticity. Different fitness activities and recreational sports are encouraged in young people since there is a tendency to cease such activities after stroke. Somatosensory rehabilitation and speech therapy should also be included. Acupuncture may be useful for chronic fatigue. Noninvasive brain stimulation (NIBS) helps the process of neuroplasticity [36].

Regarding long-term results, studies show that the beneficial results of rehabilitation programs are maintained up to 1 year after the program is finalized [37].

A more modern and practical rehabilitation method is the StrokeBack project. The rehabilitation process can be done at home and uses telemedicine. The patients first learn the exercises with the help of a physiotherapist and then practice those exercises in the comfort of his own home. The patient's progress is being monitored and then receives feedback from his caregiver. The method has multiple advantages. Patients are more motivated because they receive constant feedback, and they have the tendency to exercise more, and as a result, their quality of life improves. Another beneficial aspect is that healthcare costs are diminished due to fewer hospital visits. This program would also be helpful especially given the current situation, the Covid-19 pandemic. Patients would still continue their rehabilitation process at home for an indefinite period [38].

2.9 Prevention of stroke in young adults

Primary and secondary stroke prevention is identical both for the young and for the elderly [2]. Prevention focuses primarily on classical cardiovascular risk factors: hypertensions, dyslipidemia, and diabetes. Drug use should be actively discouraged, and a healthy lifestyle promoted: lose weight, exercise regularly, cease smoking, reduce alcohol consumption, and eat more fresh fruits and vegetables [8]. In addition, depending on the etiology, prevention should be individualized and specific measures should be taken.

Another important aspect is raising awareness regarding stroke's most common signs and symptoms. Presentation to hospitals is usually delayed because of improper identification. Patients or bystanders fail to recognize the symptoms and signs of stroke. This is due to the fact that stoke is still considered an illness affecting exclusively the elderly. As a consequence, education programs should be implemented in schools, and awareness campaigns should be created [39, 40].

3. Conclusions

Due to the increasing incidence and the possibility of it leaving long-term consequences, ischemic stroke can be considered a public health concern. Although less suspected in the young, these patients require early identification and must receive rapid medical care. For this reason, awareness campaigns should be developed. People should know that stroke can occur at any age and be aware of its most important signs and symptoms.

The etiology of ischemic stroke in the young differs from that found in the elderly. The possible causes are multiple, including rare genetic ones. But unfortunately, very often, the causes remain unidentified. One possible explanation of this phenomenon is that there are currently no specific guidelines for stroke management in young patients. For this reason, for the diagnosis, treatment, and subsequently secondary prevention of ischemic stroke, a series of universal management guidelines should be developed with priority.

Keeping in mind that stroke occurs at people of young age, with long-life spans ahead, the prognosis of patients after the ischemic event is important to be evaluated. Consequently, developing universal prognosis scores could be extremely valuable. Another particularly important aspect would be determining the risk of recurrence.

Due to increased prevalence of classic cardiovascular risk factors at younger age, physicians should also focus on primary and secondary prevention, actively counseling patients regarding these risk factors, and offer support in their attempt to gradually change their lifestyle. Patients should be advised to give up smoking, exercise regularly, lose weight, rest properly, and reduce alcohol consumption.

Such measures and initiatives should ease the diagnosis process of determining the cause of stroke in young patients, help better manage the case, and reduce the recurrence rate.

Author details

Diana Mihai[1], Florentina Cristina Plesa[1,2], Any Docu Axelerad[3,4], Alice Munteanu[5], Minerva Claudia Ghinescu[2] and Carmen Adella Sirbu[1,2]*

1 Central Military Emergency University Hospital, Department of Neurology, Bucharest, Romania

2 Titu Maiorescu University, Bucharest, Romania

3 Faculty of Medicine, 'Ovidius' University of Constanta, Department of Neurology, Romania

4 Clinical Emergency Hospital 'St. Apostol Andrei', Constanta, Romania

5 Central Military Emergency University Hospital, Department of Cardiology, Bucharest, Romania

*Address all correspondence to: sircar13@yahoo.com

References

[1] Boot E, Ekker MS, Putaala J, Kittner S, De Leeuw FE, Tuladhar AM. Ischaemic stroke in young adults: A global perspective. Journal of Neurology, Neurosurgery, and Psychiatry. 2020;**91**(4):411-417. DOI: 10.1136/jnnp-2019-322424

[2] Mehndiratta MP. Stroke in the young: Newer concepts in etiopathogenesis and risk factors. Astrocytes. 2018;**5**(1):1-4. DOI: 10.4103/2349-0977.250951

[3] Ekker MS, Boot EM, Singhal AB, et al. Epidemiology, aetiology, and management of ischaemic stroke in young adults. Lancet Neurology. 2018;**17**(9):790-801. DOI: 10.1016/S1474-4422(18)30233-3

[4] Putaala J. Ischemic stroke in the young: Current perspectives on incidence, risk factors, and cardiovascular prognosis. European Stroke Journal. 2016;**1**(1):28-40. DOI: 10.1177/2396987316629860

[5] Griffiths D, Sturm J. Epidemiology and etiology of young stroke. Stroke Research and Treatment. 2011;**2011**:209370. DOI: 10.4061/2011/209370

[6] Caplan L, Liebeskind D. Pathology, anatomy, and pathophysiology of stroke. In: Caplan L, editor. Caplan's Stroke: A Clinical Approach. Cambridge: Cambridge University Press; 2016. pp. 19-54. DOI: 10.1017/CBO9781316095805.003

[7] Easton JD, Saver JL, Albers GW. Definition and evaluation of transient ischemic attack. Stroke. 2006;**37**(1):263-266

[8] Smajlović D. Strokes in young adults: Epidemiology and prevention. Vascular Health and Risk Management. 2015;**11**:157-164. DOI: 10.2147/VHRM.S53203

[9] van Alebeek ME, de Heus R, Tuladhar AM, de Leeuw FE. Pregnancy and ischemic stroke: A practical guide to management. Current Opinion in Neurology. 2018;**31**(1):44-51. DOI: 10.1097/WCO.0000000000000522

[10] DeVeber G, Singhal A, Caplan L. Stroke in children and young adults. In: Caplan L, editor. Caplan's Stroke: A Clinical Approach. Cambridge: Cambridge University Press; 2016. pp. 511-533. DOI: 10.1017/CBO9781316095805.016

[11] Sanchetee PC, Dhamija RM, Roy AK, Venkataraman S. Peripartum cerebral venous thrombosis. The Journal of the Association of Physicians of India. 1992;**40**(10):664-666

[12] Bateman K, Bryer A. Strokes in persons infected with HIV. In: Caplan L, Biller J, editors. Uncommon Causes of Stroke. Cambridge: Cambridge University Press; 2018. pp. 52-62. DOI: 10.1017/9781316551684.009

[13] Caplan L, Amarenco P. Brain embolism. In: Caplan L, editor. Caplan's Stroke: A Clinical Approach. Cambridge: Cambridge University Press; 2016. pp. 312-363. DOI: 10.1017/CBO9781316095805.011

[14] Thaler D, Cramer S. Paradoxical embolisms and strokes. In: Caplan L, Biller J, editors. Uncommon Causes of Stroke. Cambridge: Cambridge University Press; 2018. pp. 565-574. DOI: 10.1017/9781316551684.071

[15] Engelter ST, Traenka C, Lyrer PA. Stroke caused by cervical artery dissection. In: Lee SH, editor. Stroke Revisited: Diagnosis and Treatment of Ischemic Stroke. Singapore: Stroke Revisited. Springer; 2017

[16] Arnold M, Sturzenegger M. CERVICO-cephalic arterial dissections.

In: Caplan L, Bogousslavsky J, editors. Uncommon Causes of Stroke. Cambridge: Cambridge University Press; 2008. pp. 433-454. DOI: 10.1017/CBO9780511544897.061

[17] Maria-Gabriela C, Corina R. Neurorehabilitation in basilar artery occlusion in a young patient with thrombophilia and antiphospholipid antibody syndrome – A case report. Balneo Research Journal. 2019;**10**:8-11. DOI: 10.12680/balneo.2019.231

[18] Caplan L, Biller J. Non-atherosclerotic vasculopathies. In: Caplan L, editor. Caplan's Stroke: A Clinical Approach. Cambridge: Cambridge University Press; 2016. pp. 386-438. DOI: 10.1017/CBO9781316095805.013

[19] Tatlisumak T, Putaala J, Debette S. Less common causes of stroke: Diagnosis and management. In: Oxford Textbook of Stroke and Cerebrovascular Disease. Oxford, UK: Oxford University Press; 2014. Available from: https://oxfordmedicine.com/view/10

[20] Gutierrez J, Mira K, Elkind MSV. Collagen vascular and infectious diseases. In: Stroke: Pathophysiology, Diagnosis, and Management. UK: Elsevier Inc.; 2015. pp. 619-631

[21] Lang W, Karl M. Less common stroke syndromes. Chapter. In: Michael B, Wolf-Dieter H, editors. Textbook of Stroke Medicine. 3rd ed. Cambridge: Cambridge University Press; 2019. pp. 182-201. DOI: 10.1017/9781108659574.011

[22] Sanchetee P. Stroke and central nervous system infections. Journal of the Indian Medical Association. 2009;**107**(6):372-377

[23] Klok FA, Kruip MJHA, van der Meer NJM, Arbous MS, Gommers DAMPJ, Kant KM, et al. Incidence of thrombotic complications in critically ill ICU patients with COVID-19. Thrombosis Research. 2020;**S0049-3848**(20)30120-1. DOI: 10.1016/j.thromres.2020.04.013. [published online ahead of print, 10 April 2020]

[24] Mackey J. Evaluation and management of stroke in young adults. Continuum (Minneap Minn). 2014;**20**(2 Cerebrovascular Disease):352-369. DOI: 10.1212/01.CON.0000446106.74796.e9

[25] Meschia JF, Woo D, Werring D. Genetic basis of stroke occurrence, prevention and outcome. In: Stroke: Pathophysiology, Diagnosis, and Management. UK: Elsevier Inc.; 2015. pp. 268-279. DOI: 10.1016/B978-0-323-29544-4.00018-9

[26] Choi JC. Genetic causes of ischemic stroke. In: Lee SH, editor. Stroke Revisited: Diagnosis and Treatment of Ischemic Stroke. Singapore: Stroke Revisited. Springer; 2017

[27] Lynch DS, Wade C, ARB P, et al. Practical approach to the diagnosis of adult-onset leukodystrophies: An updated guide in the genomic era. Journal of Neurology, Neurosurgery, and Psychiatry. 2019;**90**(5):543-554. DOI: 10.1136/jnnp-2018-319481

[28] Caplan L, Bousser M. Cerebral venous thrombosis. In: Caplan L, editor. Caplan's Stroke: A Clinical Approach. Cambridge: Cambridge University Press; 2016. pp. 544-566. DOI: 10.1017/CBO9781316095805.018

[29] B K. Cerebral Venous Sinus Thrombosis. 2017. DOI: 10.1007/978-981-10-1424-6_16

[30] Bhatt N, Malik AM, Chaturvedi S. Stroke in young adults: Five new things. Neurology Clinical Practice. 2018;**8**(6):501-506. DOI: 10.1212/CPJ.0000000000000522

[31] Al Khathaami AM, Alsaif SA, Al Bdah BA, et al. Stroke mimics:

Clinical characteristics and outcome. Neurosciences (Riyadh). 2020;**25**(1):38-42. DOI: 10.17712/nsj.2020.1.20190096

[32] Vilela, P. Acute stroke differential diagnosis: Stroke mimics. European Journal of Radiology. 2017;**96**:133-144. DOI: 10.1016/j.ejrad.2017.05.008

[33] Papavasileiou V, Goldstein LB. Thrombolysis in young adults with acute ischemic stroke: Quicker may be better. Neurology. 2019;**92**(24):1129-1130. DOI: 10.1212/WNL.0000000000007651

[34] Teasell R, Foley N, Hussein N, Cotoi A. The Efficacy of Stroke Rehabilitation in Evidence Based Review of Stroke Rehabilitation. 18th ed. Ontario, Canada: EBRSR; 2018

[35] Cotoi A, Batey C, Hussein N, Janzen S, Teasell R. Rehabilitation of Younger Patients Post Stroke in Evidence Based Review of Stroke Rehabilitation. 18th ed. Ontario, Canada: EBRSR; 2018

[36] Brainin M, Heiss W, editors. Therapeutic strategies and neurorehabilitation. In: Textbook of Stroke Medicine. Cambridge: Cambridge University Press; 2014. pp. 285-398. DOI: 10.1017/CBO9781107239340.018

[37] Teasell R, Foley N, Hussein N, Wiener J, Speechley M. The Elements of Stroke Rehabilitation in Evidence Based Review of Stroke Rehabilitation. 18th ed2018

[38] Vogiatzaki E, Krukowski A. Motivation, market and european perspective. In: Vogiatzaki E, Krukowski A, editors. Modern Stroke Rehabilitation through e-Health-Based Entertainment. Cham: Springer; 2016. DOI: 10.1007/978-3-319-21293-7_1

[39] Singhal AB, Biller J, Elkind MS, et al. Recognition and management of stroke in young adults and adolescents. Neurology. 2013;**81**(12):1089-1097. DOI: 10.1212/WNL.0b013e3182a4a451

[40] Amey V, Jing Z, Renyu L. Too Young to Have a Stroke?—a Global Health Crisis. Stroke and Vascular Neurology. 2019;**4**:173-175. DOI: 10.1136/svn-2019-000295

Chapter 3

Vascular Aphasias

Dragoș Cătălin Jianu, Silviana Nina Jianu, Ligia Petrica, Traian Flavius Dan and Georgiana Munteanu

Abstract

Aphasia represents an acquired central disorder of language that impairs a person's ability to understand and/or produce spoken and written language, caused by lesions situated usually in the dominant (left) cerebral hemisphere, in right-handed persons. Aphasia has a prevalence of 25–30% in acute ischemic stroke (vascular aphasia). It is considered as an important stroke severity marker, being associated with a higher risk of mortality, poor functional prognosis, and augmented risk of vascular dementia. The assessment of aphasias in clinical practice is based on classical analysis of oral production and comprehension. The language disturbances are frequently combined into aphasic syndromes which are components of different vascular syndromes that may evolve/involve rapidly at the acute stage of ischemic stroke. The main determinant of the type of vascular aphasia is the infarct location (especially left middle cerebral artery territory). Recent studies at the hyperacute stage of ischemic stroke have observed features of aphasia, have reanalyzed its neuroanatomy using new imaging techniques, and have shown that aphasias have a parallel course to that of cortico-subcortical hypoperfusion. Thus, the reversal of hypoperfusion, following recanalization (spontaneous or secondary to thrombolysis or thrombectomy), is associated with resolution of aphasia. Speech therapy is needed as soon as permitted by clinical condition.

Keywords: language, speech, aphasia, vascular aphasia, hyperacute stage of ischemic stroke, language therapy

1. Introduction

Aphasia is one of the most common and also frustrating disabilities secondary to stroke; over 25% of the patients who suffer an acute ischemic stroke are dealing with this complex syndrome in their evolution. It is also considered an important stroke severity marker, being associated with a higher risk of mortality, poor functional prognosis, and augmented risk of vascular dementia. This syndrome is a real challenge not only for the patients or their relatives but also for the specialists (neurologists, speech therapists, psychologists, and physiotherapists) involved in the diagnosis and treatment of those patients.

The assessment of aphasias in clinical practice is based on classical analysis of oral production and comprehension. The language disturbances are frequently combined into aphasic syndromes (nonfluent/fluent aphasias), which are constituents of different vascular syndromes, being accompanied by motor deficit of the right limbs or visual deficit (hemianopia). The main determinant of the type of vascular aphasia is the infarct location (especially left middle cerebral artery territory). Recent studies at the hyperacute stage of ischemic stroke have observed features of aphasia, have reanalyzed its neuroanatomy using new imaging techniques, and have shown that aphasias have a parallel course to that of cortico-subcortical hypoperfusion. Thus, the reversal of hypoperfusion, following recanalization (spontaneous or secondary to thrombolysis or thrombectomy), is associated with resolution of aphasia. Speech therapy is needed as soon as permitted by clinical condition. Unfortunately, pharmacotherapy remains to be evaluated. Other studies examined the potential interest of new treatment, such as transcranial magnetic stimulation.

This chapter is meant to clarify different aspects regarding the definition, classification, diagnosis criteria, and therapeutically strategies for the most common vascular aphasic syndromes due to ischemic stroke.

2. Language and speech

In the field of neurolinguistics, there are two words, often misused as synonyms: "language" and "speech," although each one of these terms describes different functions regarding distinct processes and involving distinct neural networks [1].

Language is a noninstinctive, culturally driven system of voluntarily produced symbols, involving receptive and expressive skills enabling understanding and expression of information or emotion. It represents a complex interaction between sensory-motor abilities and symbolic combinations, so that people can communicate [1].

The language system consists of five domains [1]:

1. *Phonology*: The systematic organization of different sounds in spoken languages and linguistic rules of their pronunciation and perception. It is different from phonetics. While phonology reveals the modality sounds come together within a certain language to encode meaning (to form words), phonetics describes the physical production, acoustic transmission, and perception of the sounds of speech.

2. *Morphology*: The study of the internal structure of words, how they are formed, and their relationship to other words in the same language. Morphemes represent the minimal units of words that have meaning and, in the same time, cannot be subdivided further (free morphemes can appear alone: example: "good," but bound morphemes: example: "ly" must be added to a free morpheme to produce a word).

3. *Semantics*: The systematic meaning of words represents the study of relations between words and what they denote; it means the signification of words reflecting content and utterance intent.

4. *Syntax*: The set of linguistic principles that define the way in which words order ("arrange together") to convey a complete thought, and to form correct sentences or phrases in a given language: example: the sequence in which the subject (S), verb (V), and object (O) combine in sentences: usually in the sequence SVO or SOV.

5. *Pragmatics*: The rules for maintaining a conversation in terms of responsiveness and relevance. It defines the way people produce and comprehend intended meanings through language, in actual situations. Unlike semantics, which defines meaning that is conventional (grammar and lexicon) in a given language, pragmatics explains how the speaker and listener are capable to overcome apparent ambiguity in a peculiar context.

Speech results from the extremely coordinated rapid motor functions, thereby requiring the combination of phonation (voicing), resonance (nasality), articulation, fluency, and prosody. It is responsible for the actual act of vocal expression of language. The most important neural structures involved in the regulation of speech are represented by the cortical systems, the basal ganglia, the cerebellum, and the corticobulbar tracts, via the nuclei of the trigeminal, facial, glossopharyngeal, vagal, accessory (spinal), hypoglossal, and phrenic nerves. All these structures maintain the control and coordination between all the muscles involved in speaking: oral, lingual, palatal, pharyngeal, laryngeal, and respiratory muscles [1].

3. Definition of aphasia

Aphasia represents an acquired central disorder of language that impairs a person's ability to understand or/and produce spoken language, often associated with impairment in reading (alexia) and writing (agraphia). Aphasia may supplementary affect the person's ability to use musical notation, mathematical operations, etc.; in consequence, the aphasic may present difficulties to generate and use symbol systems. Aphasia is different from a peripheral (sensory-motor) disorder of language that may mimic aphasia (such as weakness of the muscles of articulation). In the same time, it is an acquired phenomenon that appears after the language has already been learned [1–4].

4. Language localization

Nowadays, in the era of functional neuroimaging, using a variety of complex techniques, organization of the language network has been partially understood. The outward production of language is the effect of neural activation in huge network including different regions in the cortex, basal ganglia, cerebellum, and brainstem. An overlap in that network or with other networks of specialization determines the huge clinical spectrum following an acquired injury. One lesion in an area can produce numerous signs, and injuries concerning distinct areas can result in similar deficits [1].

Functional neuroimaging studies mentioned that the "language network" is strikingly similar across different language tasks and across different healthy people: *the dorsal frontoparietal pathway*—for articulatory and syntactic processes and *the ventral temporal pathway*—for mapping sounds to lexical representations and meanings of words [1].

Aphasia is caused by a localized brain damage. Using a combination of different neuroimaging techniques, it has been suggested that *core language functions are perisylvian left—lateralized regions* in the majority of patients (95% right-handers and 75% left-handers, respectively) [1]. These regions include (a) *anterior areas* and (b) *posterior areas* [1–5]:

Anterior areas	Posterior areas
• The Broca's area: the posterior part of the third frontal gyrus-F3 (Brodmann areas: BA 44 and 45) • The Rolandic operculum (lower part of the motor area: Fa) • The insular cortex and the subjacent white matter • The left premotor and prefrontal regions (situated anterior and superior of Broca's area) • The supplementary motor area	• The Wernicke's area: the posterior part of the first two temporal gyri-T1/T2 (BA 22) • The inferior parietal lobes: the angular gyrus (BA 39), and the supramarginal gyrus (BA 40) • The anterior part of the temporal lobe

Recent studies [2], using MRI, noted the following correlations between different linguistic disturbances and cerebral lesions due to ischemic strokes:

• Reduction in fluency of spontaneous speech • Impaired repetition • Oral comprehension • Anomia (naming deficits)	• Inferior frontal gyrus • Putamen • Anterior subcortical lesions • Insular and external and posterior internal lesions • The posterior part of the superior and middle temporal gyri • The external capsule • The insula and the inferior frontal gyrus • Insula and external capsule • Posterior subcortical • Head of caudate nucleus • Medial temporal, middle and inferior frontal gyri, and genu of internal capsule

5. The evaluation of language disturbances

The assessment of aphasias in clinical practice is based on the analysis of six different language domains, which are represented by oral production (expressive language), comprehension (language understanding), repetition, naming, reading, and writing (**Figure 1**) [1–6].

5.1 Assessment of oral production (expressive language/spontaneous speech)

It refers to modifications of fluency, prosody and volume, and presence of deviations at various linguistic levels [1–7].

Fluency is represented by the flow of speech (number of words per minute: wpm) and effort (smoothness).

The main deviations at different linguistic levels of oral production are as follows:

a. *Sound/articulation level* (incorrect articulation of a sound): dysarthria

b. *Phonemic level* (addition, omission, substitution, or inversion of a phoneme): phonological paraphasias

c. *Verbal level* (word-selection/lexicon): word-finding difficulties (anomia), are the core symptom of aphasias, usually associated with verbal (semantic) paraphasias, perseveration, circumlocutions, or, even, neologisms

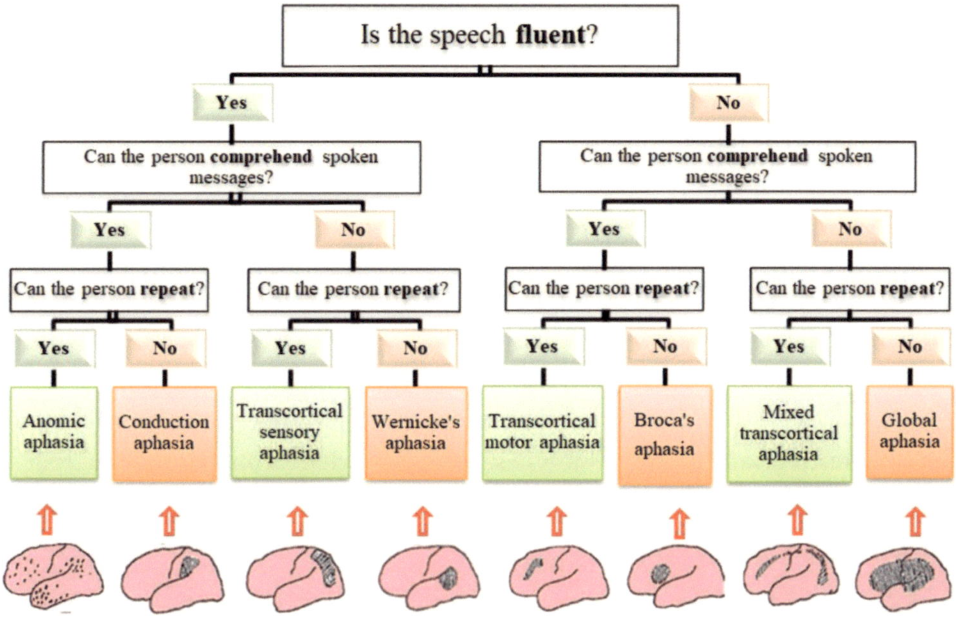

Figure 1.
The assessment of aphasias in clinical practice is based on the classical analysis of oral production (fluency), comprehension, and repetition.

d. *Syntactic level* (grammar): agrammatism characterized by a severe diminution in the use of grammatical elements in language (in Broca's aphasia), and paragrammatism with an overuse of wrongly selected grammatical elements (in Wernicke's aphasia)

Other deviations are represented by oral production restricted to a few stereotyped utterances (e.g., "tan tan"), jargon aphasia (associating frequently multiple phonemic and verbal deviations leading to neologisms), echolalia, and the "conduit d'approche" (i.e., numerous attempts to correct phonemic deformations by successive approximations).

There are two types of aphasias: nonfluent (Broca's aphasia, transcortical motor aphasia, and global aphasia) and fluent (Wernicke's aphasia, transcortical sensory aphasia, and conduction aphasia). On the one hand, a nonfluent spontaneous speech presents less than 50 wpm, augmented effort, dysprosodia, sometimes hypophonia, dysarthria, few paraphasias (especially phonological paraphasias), substantive words in excess, and short sentences. On the other hand, a fluent speech presents a normal of words per minute (100–200 wpm), with a normal effort, normal prosody and volume, no deviation at sound level (correct articulation of a sound), many paraphasias (including verbal paraphasias), relatively lack of substantive words, and normal sentences (including 5–8 wps) [1–7].

5.2 Assessment of oral comprehension

It analyses comprehension at the linguistic levels of word and syntax [1–7]. Oral comprehension is formally examined by (a) asking the aphasic to point an object, a body part, etc. and (b) presenting different verbal commands with augmenting complexity. Impaired oral comprehension is usually underdiagnosed in clinical practice. We should think at this language disturbance when a patient does not behave according to the examiner's tasks, especially during object pointing on verbal command and tasks using sentences of progressive complexity. The shortened Token Test is the test usually used to exam if the comprehension is impaired (adjusted score <29) and to differentiate Broca from global aphasia (adjusted score <17) [2, 6].

5.3 Assessment of repetition

When testing repetition, it is essential to use different types of items (short-long verbal information and meaningful-meaningless utterances) [1–7].

Aphasias with impaired repetition ability (perisylvian aphasias) differ from this point of view from transcortical (extrasylvian) aphasias, with normal repetition (even if oral comprehension is severely impaired in transcortical sensory aphasia).

5.4 Naming

While testing naming, different types should be included: objects, body parts, actions, and colors ("What is this?") [5–7]. If we want to assess the understanding ability of the patient, we have to exam pointing ("Show me, please, where the...is!"), which is the opposite of naming [5, 6].

5.5 Reading (lexia)

While testing reading, we should focus on two aspects: (a) the mechanisms of reading (the conversion of visual signs-graphemes into phonemes) and (b) reading comprehension (using written commands, etc.) [5–7].

5.6 Writing (graphia)

We should exam spontaneous writing, writing by dictation, and copying at different levels of the writing language: letters, syllables, words, sentences, and texts [5–7].

The different language disturbances observed are frequently combined into aphasic syndromes (nonfluent/fluent aphasias) [1, 2, 5, 7].

An experimented examiner can diagnose the aphasic syndrome based on analysis of six language domains (oral production, etc.).

However, clinical examination can produce two kinds of errors: (a) underestimation of oral comprehension deficit and (b) misdiagnose of verbal stereotypies with jargon aphasia.

These errors are not found in the case of assessment of aphasias using an aphasia battery test:

- Boston Diagnostic Aphasia Examination (BDAE) [8]
- Western Aphasia Battery (WAB) [9]
- Montreal-Toulouse Language Assessment Battery [10]
- Minnesota Test for Differential Diagnosis of Aphasia [6]
- Multilingual Aphasia Examination [6]
- Bilingual Aphasia Test [6]

Each test provides well-defined cut-off scores, so the description of the aphasic syndrome is more precise than that obtained on clinical grounds [2].

Bilingual Aphasia Test (BAT) [6] was realized to exam each of the languages of a bilingual or polyglot aphasic in an equivalent way. The test is available in dozens of different pairs of languages. Thus, the various versions of the BAT are linguistically equivalent tests [6].

6. Types of aphasic syndromes

The main determinants of the type of aphasias are *the site* and *size of the lesion* [2]. In the same time, *age* (with a higher frequency of nonfluent aphasias in young patients) and *sex* (with a higher frequency of nonfluent aphasias in men) are two other determinants. This aspect has been observed only in aphasics with ischemic stroke, but not in those with hemorrhagic stroke or tumors [2, 11].

Types of aphasic syndromes (nonfluent/fluent aphasias) [1, 2, 8] are:

1. Broca's aphasia

2. Wernicke's aphasia

3. Conduction aphasia

4. Transcortical aphasias:

    a. Transcortical motor aphasia

    b. Transcortical sensory aphasia

    c. Mixed transcortical aphasia

5. Global aphasias

6. Anomic plus aphasias

The global aphasia (24–38%) and anomic plus aphasia (20%) are more frequent in acute ischemic stroke; Broca (10–15%), Wernicke (15%), and transcortical motor aphasias (15–20%) present an intermediate frequency, and other aphasias are rare [1, 2, 5].

About 10% of aphasias remain unclassifiable, especially in patients with a previous ischemic stroke (atypical aphasias: mixed aphasias, thalamic aphasias, and capsulo-striatal aphasias) [2, 12–14].

6.1 Broca's aphasia

6.1.1 Clinical aspects

A. Assessment of oral production (spontaneous speech)

1. Fluency

When there is no aphasic mutism or when mutism has regressed, the patient presents a nonfluent, arduous verbal output, characterized by difficulties to initiate spontaneous speech, effortful with hesitations and slow output (10–15 words/minute), and interrupted by word-finding pauses. Sometimes, he presents dysprosody (oral expression is monotonously, melodic modulation being absent) [1–5, 15–18].

2. Presence of deviations at various levels

    a. Sound/arthric level (incorrect articulation of a sound)—dysarthria.

    b. Phonemic level (omission, substitution, addition, or inversion of a phoneme)—phonemic paraphasias.

    c. Verbal level (naming): semantic (verbal) paraphasias; word-finding difficulty (anomia), especially in spontaneous speech; deficits in action naming are more severe than deficits in object naming.

    d. Syntactic level: agrammatism, usually more apparent after the acute phase: omission of functional/grammatical words (prepositions, conjunctions, articles, auxiliary verbs/e.g. "the," "an," and inflections), while conceptual words (nouns, verbs, and adverbs) are used in a greater proportion—"telegraphic speech." Sometimes, the oral production can be restricted to a few stereotyped utterances (e.g., "tan tan") [4, 5, 17, 19].

B. Assessment of repetition

Poor repetition—The patient will find difficult to repeat operational words and flexional endings, resulting phonemic and verbal paraphasias (e.g., "The boy eats an apple"/"Boy-eat-apple"). Repetition and naming are impaired, although this is less marked than spontaneous speech.

Automatic speech—Enumerating the days of the week, the months of the year, numbering from 1 to 10, repeating a poem, and so on, can ameliorate the verbal output [17, 20, 21].

C. Assessment of oral comprehension

Usually, good oral comprehension, at least for commands, is needed to permit clinical exam. In some cases, syntactic comprehension can be affected as requested to understand complex sentences and multiple instructions [2]:

a. The patient is unable to distinguish between different operational words like "on" or "in."

b. Comprehension of passive reversible sentences can be affected [18, 22].

Example:
(Q): "The girl was kissed by the boy. Who kissed whom?
(A): Girl kiss boy."

D. Assessment of reading and writing

Reading (frontal alexia-literal alexia) and writing (frontal agraphia) are also impaired [20].

In conclusion, three characteristics represent the core of Broca's aphasia: dysarthria, agrammatism, and preserved comprehension [1–5].

6.1.2 Associated signs and symptoms

1. Contralateral hemiparesis—lesions that cause Broca's aphasia also interrupt adjacent cortical motor fibers and deep fiber tracts.

2. Facial weakness.

3. Buccofacial apraxia/apraxia of speech, which represents a disturbance in motor programming of speech articulation. The patient is aware of his deficit, so he tries unsuccessfully to correct his disturbance by trial and error. Instead, he presents difficulty in initiating utterances, groping articulatory movements, and articulatory inconsistency on repeated attempts of the same utterance.

4. The patient with Broca's aphasia is aware of his oral expression disorders; consequently, he can develop depression [1–3].

6.1.3 Anatomo-clinical correlations

Lesions or dysfunctions usually involves on the left side in right-handed individuals (**Figure 2**):

a. Broca's area: the posterior part of the third frontal gyrus-Brodmann areas 44 and 45.

Lesions in this area determine transitory apraxia of speech. Larger lesions, involving Broca's area and its subjacent white matter, produce transitory mutism, which is replaced by a rapidly improving syndrome with prominent arthric deformations and deficits in action naming that are more severe than deficits in object naming.

b. Rolandic operculum: lower part of motor area: Fa.

c. Lesions can extend or separately affect insular cortex, and subjacent white matter, centrum semiovale, capsulostriatum (caudate nucleus head and putamen), and periventricular areas. Infarctions involving together these structures and Broca's area can produce the complete syndrome of Broca's aphasia.

Broca's aphasia is produced by infarcts/severe hypoperfusion (MRI of the brain) of the superior division of the left MCA [1, 2, 5, 23–25].

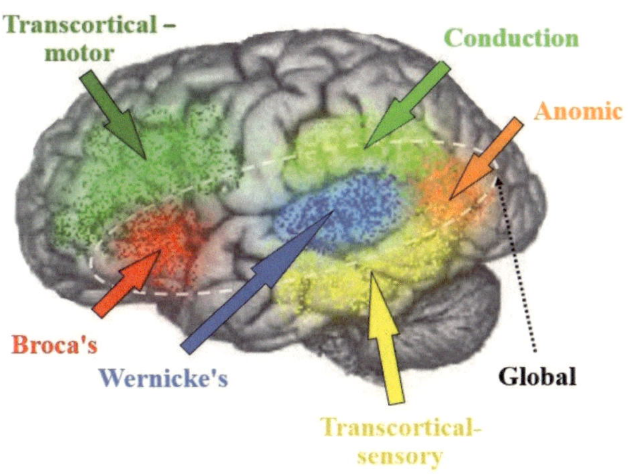

Figure 2.
Different types of aphasias: anatomo-clinical correlations.

6.2 Wernicke's aphasia

6.2.1 Clinical aspects

A. Assessment of oral production (spontaneous speech)

1. Fluency

The verbal output is fluent, with easy initialization of speech, plentiful output (100–200 words/minute), the phrase length is normal (~5–8 words/phrase), with normal prosody. There is no quantitative reduction of spontaneous speech. In some cases, the oral production may be augmented (logorrhea), concerning patients with jargon aphasia and anosognosia (differential diagnosis with acute delirium) [1, 2, 5, 26–28].

2. Presence of deviations at various levels:

a. Sound/arthric level: good articulation of sounds, well-articulated speech

b. Phonemic level: verbal paraphasias (semantically related word substitutions), phonemic paraphasias (phonologically related word or nonword substitutions), and jargon aphasia (associating frequently multiple paraphasias leading to neologisms)

c. Verbal level (naming): word-finding difficulty anomia (naming is severely affected), frequently associated circumlocutions, perseveration, and occasional neologisms

d. Syntactic level: paragrammatism: nouns replaced by pronouns ("that" and "those") or by unspecific words ("thing" and "something") [1, 2, 5, 26–28]

B. Assessment of repetition

Repetition is severely impaired [1, 2, 5, 26–28].

C. Assessment of oral comprehension

Oral comprehension is severe impaired, due to disturbances in language sounds perception (repetition is impossible); incapacity of accessing the meaning of the word (repetition is normal); decrease in verbal memory (repetition may be disturbed depending on the length of the verbal output of the speaker); perturbation in comprehension of the lexicosemantic relations of the phrase or utterance [1, 2, 5, 26–28].

Sometimes, comprehension is more difficult for isolated words; on the other hand, verbal reception of some lexicosemantic categories may be partially or totally preserved. Syntactic comprehension is significant affected [1, 2, 5, 26–28].

D. Assessment of reading and writing

Reading is frequently impaired (alexia).

Writing (agraphia): spontaneous and dictated writing are fully of paragraphia and paragrammatism; copying a text is easier than writing after hearing one [1, 2, 5, 26–28].

6.2.2 Associated signs and symptoms

1. Homonymous hemianopia—frequently associated.

2. Complete/dissociated Gerstmann syndrome (agraphia, acalculia, finger agnosia, and inability to distinguish between the right and left sides of one's body).

3. Limb apraxia.

4. Anosognosia—it can be observed at the initial stage and decreases gradually; high excitation: logorrhea and exaggeration of mimico-gestural language. The patient with Wernicke's aphasia, in contrast to a Broca's aphasic, is unaware of his disorders and seems unconcerned [1, 2, 5, 26–28].

6.2.3 Anatomo-clinical correlations

a. Wernicke's area: posterior part of the first two temporal gyri-T1/T2 (BA 22) (**Figure** 2).

b. Inferior parietal lobes: angular gyrus (BA 39) and supramarginal gyrus (BA 40).

c. Lesions can extend to the insular-external capsule region and anterior part of temporal gyri (BA22). Besides the cortical destructions from these areas, subjacent white matter can be also affected.

Wernicke's aphasia is the result of an infarct/sever hypoperfusion (MRI of the brain) of the inferior division of the left MCA (supplies the posterior part of the temporal lobe and inferior parietal lobule), usually an embolic occlusion/atherothrombotic [1, 2, 5, 23–25].

Wernicke's aphasia is more current in elderly women, due to a higher frequency of infarct in the inferior-posterior territory of the MCA in these patients [1, 2, 5].

6.3 Conduction aphasia

6.3.1 Clinical aspects

A. Assessment of oral production (spontaneous speech)

1. Fluency: verbal output (spontaneous speech) is fluent, although some hesitations and self-correction attempts to interrupt the flow are noted [1, 2, 5, 29–32].

2. Presence of deviations at various levels

   a. Sound/arthric level: normal articulation (speech well-articulated).

   b. Phonemic level: phonemic paraphasias are typically for conduction aphasia. The production of phonemic paraphasias across verbal tasks represents the cardinal feature of conduction aphasia.

   - Semantic/verbal paraphasias or neologisms are less frequent in conduction aphasia than in other fluent types of aphasia.

c. Verbal level (naming): anomia—naming may be mildly impaired.

d. Syntactic level: the grammar is preserved. Sentences are short and have simple syntax [1, 2, 5, 29–32].

B. Assessment of repetition

Repetition is impaired, contrasting with the sparing of the oral comprehension. Repetition of monosyllabic or bisyllabic words can be normal, but repetition of polysyllabic words and of sentences is always incorrect. The patient often paraphrases the sentence rather than repeating it.

Repetitive self-corrections, word-finding difficulties, and paraphrasing are attempts to correct phonemic deformations by successive approximations, named "conduit d'approche" [2, 29–32].

C. Assessment of oral comprehension

It involves sparing of oral comprehension. The patient understands simple, active sentences, but guesses at comprehension of passive sentences [1, 2, 5, 29–32].

D. Assessment of reading and writing

It involves usually good reading comprehension, but paraphasic oral reading. More precisely, the patient has difficulties in spelling and reading unfamiliar words, but correctly reads and spells words.

In conclusion, conduction aphasia presents three major characteristics: a relatively fluent, though phonologically paraphasic speech; poor repetition; and relatively spared comprehension [1, 2, 5, 29–32].

6.3.2 Associated signs and symptoms

1. Oral and limb apraxia; ideomotor apraxia

2. Right sensory impairment [1, 2, 5]

6.3.3 Anatomo-clinical correlations

The lesions affect the inferior parietal lobes, especially the supramarginal gyrus or/and the external capsule; they classically disrupt the arcuate fasciculus (a large bundle of fibers), although its role remains debated for the repetition impairments: probably disconnection between the superior temporal cortex and the inferior frontal gyri, respectively (**Figure 2**).

Other explanations for the repetition impairments have been noted, such as short-term memory syndrome (the repetition impairment due to limited working memory)—so, the associated lesions are situated in areas critical for working memory: inferior parietal lobule (supramarginal and angular gyri), inferior frontal cortex, posterior temporal lobe, and/or their white matter connections (the external capsule).

Conduction aphasia is the result of an embolic infarct of the inferior division (posterior temporal or parietal) of the left MCA [1, 2, 5, 23–25].

It is rarely observed at the acute stage of stroke and more frequently affects younger patients.

6.4 Transcortical aphasias

Transcortical aphasias are the less common type of aphasias. They are characterized by preservation of word repetition, even of those words without meaning. Repetition of words is mediated by the perisylvian cerebral region (fronto-temporo-parietal region). Generally, in this type of aphasia, Broca's area, Wernicke's area, and the arcuate fasciculus are intact. In transcortical aphasia exists a disconnection between motor and/or sensory areas of language from hemispheric cortex, a process that occurs from lesions of border areas: (a) from ACA and MCA (transcortical motor aphasia) and (b) from MCA and PCA (transcortical sensory aphasia) [1, 2, 23–25].

6.4.1 Transcortical motor aphasia

6.4.1.1 Clinical aspects

It is characterized by poor spontaneous speech (nonfluent, reduced oral output with possible initial mutism, loss of initiation, hypophonia, perseveration, and reduced phrase length). Minor dysarthria is noted in opposition with sever arthric deformation noted in Broca's aphasia. Sometimes, simplification of grammatical form is noted. Echolalia and perseveration are usually observed. Naming is frequently preserved.

Repetition and oral comprehension are typically spared [1, 2, 5, 33–36].

6.4.1.1.1 Anatomo-clinical correlations

1. Cortical frontal lesions of border areas (watershed area) between the left anterior cerebral artery (ACA) and middle cerebral artery (MCA); less frequently left premotor and prefrontal regions, situated anterior and superior of Broca's area (dorsolateral region-sparing Broca area), and supplementary motor area (supero-medial area of the frontal lobe) (**Figure 2**)

2. Subcortical frontal lesions: thalamus, centrum semiovale with variable extension into the striatum (hypophonia is noted) [1, 2, 5, 23–25]

6.4.2 Transcortical sensory aphasia

6.4.2.1 Clinical aspects

Spontaneous speech (oral output) is fluent, with verbal paraphasias, word-finding difficulty (especially by naming infrequent objects and animals), and circumlocutory speech (use of generic words such as "bird" for a hen and "furniture" for a showcase).

Comprehension is severely impaired at the word level, especially for unusual nouns. This contrasts with repetition sparing (this is the key feature that distinguishes it from Wernicke's aphasia). The patient is incapable to describe accurately a name that is correctly repeated. The comprehension deficit is usually associated with semantic impairment [1, 2, 5, 33–36].

6.4.2.2 Anatomo-clinical correlations

1. Cortical lesions of border areas from MCA and posterior cerebral artery (PCA) territories: temporo-parieto-occipital junction region and inferotemporal region (second and third temporal gyri) (**Figure 2**)

2. Subcortical lesions: anterolateral thalamus

Alzheimer's disease, semantic variant of primary progressive aphasia (PPA) or Creutzfeldt-Jakob disease can produce a similar syndrome [1, 2, 5, 23–25].

6.4.3 Mixed transcortical aphasia (isolation aphasia)

6.4.3.1 Clinical aspects

Nonfluent reduced spontaneous speech (verbal output), palilalia, or even transitory mutism, combined with impaired comprehension, impaired reading (alexia), and impaired writing (agraphia), relatively spared repetition. It combines signs of both transcortical motor and sensory aphasia. It looks like a global aphasia with relatively normal repetition [1, 2, 5, 33–36].

6.4.3.1.1 Anatomo-clinical correlations

1. Cortical lesions isolating the spared perisylvian language areas (watershed territory between the left ACA and MCA in addition to the watershed territory between the left MCA and PCA) (**Figure 2**)

2. Subcortical lesions: large thalamic hemorrhage interrupting the temporal isthmus; infarcts in the left thalamus, putamen, and periventricular white matter [1, 2, 5, 23–25]

6.5 Global aphasia

6.5.1 Clinical aspects

It is the most severe form of aphasia, which associates with the following:

a. Major disorders of oral production, represented by aphasic mutism (oral output lost), or by a spontaneous speech restricted to some stereotyped utterances (with dysarthria). Repetition is severely affected (it does not improve oral output, differing from mixed transcortical aphasia).

b. Major disorders of the oral and written comprehension. Global aphasia differs from Broca's aphasia by the severity of oral comprehension impairment [1, 2, 5, 37].

6.5.1.1 Associated signs and symptoms

Right hemiparesis/hemiplegia, right hemi-hypoesthesia, right homonym hemianopia, limbs apraxia, and facio-buccolingual apraxia [1, 2, 5, 37].

6.5.1.2 Anatomo-clinical correlations

1. Extended lesions (including left perisylvian anterior and posterior language areas), which are the result of a left MCA/C1 occlusion (with a total left MCA infarct), produce global aphasia with hemiplegia, hemisensory deficits, and hemianopia (**Figure 2**) [2].

2. Broca's and Wernicke's areas may be simultaneously hypoperfused in the acute period. Thus, global aphasia can be the initial aphasic syndrome.

Early involution into Broca's aphasia (with early recovery of comprehension) may result from reperfusion of Wernicke's area. In this case, the patient presents only left frontal lobe, left basal ganglia, and left insula ischemic lesions (diffusion-weighted image shows infarct in superior division of left MCA territory, which includes Broca's area), sparing in the same time the left temporoparietal region (global aphasia with hemiplegia and early improvement of comprehension).

Later recovery of comprehension may appear from the reorganization of the language network:

3. Frontal and temporoparietal lesions (two lesions) produce global aphasia without hemiplegia. When sensory-motor deficit is missing, we should search for mixed transcortical aphasia.

4. Subcortical infarct extended into basal ganglia [1, 2, 5, 23–25, 38].

6.6 Anomic aphasia

6.6.1 Clinical aspects

Typical anomic aphasia is a fluent aphasia with word-finding difficulty anomia (noted in spontaneous speech and naming), usually associated with circumlocutions. Comprehension and repetition are spared.

Anomic plus aphasia presents additional minimal deficit of language (mild arthric deformation or mild impairment of oral comprehension or repetition). It is the mildest aphasic syndrome [1, 2, 5, 39].

6.6.2 Anatomo-clinical correlations

Acute anomic aphasia may be noted after stroke in many locations. It also represents a stage of all aphasic syndromes when they improve (**Figure 2**) [1, 2, 5, 23–25].

6.7 Peculiar aphasic syndromes

6.7.1 Crossed aphasias

This is a very rare condition (1% of all acute ischemic stroke aphasias) [39], defined by an aphasic syndrome in a right-handed patient (free from developmental disorders and previous brain lesions, fully lateralized, which is demonstrated using a questionnaire like Edinburgh Inventory) [40], caused by a right hemisphere lesion (nondominant hemisphere).

The anatomical determinants are similar to those observed in left hemisphere lesion, although a higher proportion of deviant cases are observed, particularly with mild aphasia contrasting with the large lesion. This fact is usually reported as evidence for bilateral representation of the language [2].

In the past, crossed aphasia was considered to be nonfluent, although today is reported that all aphasic syndromes can be registered (some cases of crossed Wernicke's aphasia in right-handed patients with lesions in the homologous area of the right cerebral hemisphere are noted [2].

6.7.2 Subcortical aphasias

Pure left striatocapsular infarcts (left deep MCA infarcts) can produce different types of aphasias (mainly nonfluent, especially motor transcortical aphasia and Broca's aphasia). Frequently, hypophonia (poor speech volume) can be noted.

Fluent and nonfluent aphasias have been reported in thalamic lesions. Usually, a thalamic aphasia presents a significant impairment of spontaneous speech, with verbal paraphasias, but with oral comprehension and repetition relatively spared [1, 2, 5, 28]. Patients with subcortical aphasias are older, because the main mechanism of ischemic stroke is small vascular disease.

There are two distinct mechanisms concerning subcortical vascular aphasias: (a) a possible sustained cortical hypoperfusion and infarction not visible on structural imaging studies and (b) a possible thalamic disconnection, due to striatocapsular infarcts [28].

7. Etiology of aphasias

Any type of lesion (localized/diffuse, acute/chronic, intermittent, progressive, or permanent) restricted to any of all mentioned language network from the dominant hemisphere in right-handed subjects (and rarely, in the nondominant hemisphere in right-handed subjects—"crossed aphasia") can cause aphasia [1, 2].

The most common causes of aphasia are the vascular pathology (ischemic and hemorrhagic stroke, aneurysm, cerebral veins, and dural sinus thrombosis), which produces vascular aphasias, traumatic brain injury, brain tumors, neuroinfections (especially Herpes simplex encephalitis), stroke mimics (aura migraine, epilepsy - ictal EEG sustaining the diagnosis of an epileptic seizure, and MRI-DWI), multiple sclerosis (rarely), and neurodegenerative diseases such as Alzheimer disease and primary progressive aphasia.

7.1 Vascular aphasias

Aphasia has a prevalence of 25–30% in acute ischemic stroke; it is a marker of stroke severity and of poststroke outcome, being associated with a higher risk of mortality, poor functional prognosis (can have a dramatic impact on person's ability to communicate), and increased risk of poststroke dementia [1, 2, 7–11, 41–43].

Vascular aphasias have not typically corresponded to linguistic domains network due to the fact that ischemic injuries specifically imply arterial territories, rather than being limited to the language network. Thus, the arterial syndromes include different concomitant neurological signs (hemiparesis, hemianopia, etc.,) that are reported together with aphasia because they all represent functions that depend on arterial supply of a peculiar brain region (vessel which can be occluded, producing an ischemic stroke) [1, 22, 44].

The main determinant of the type of vascular aphasia is the infarct location [1, 2]. Recent studies concerning the hyperacute stage of ischemic stroke have demonstrated that aphasic symptoms have a similar evolution to that of cortical hypoperfusion; thus, improvement in cortical perfusion (following spontaneous or therapeutic recanalization) generates recovery of aphasia [1, 2, 5, 28]. Recanalization of an occluded M1 branch of MCA through development of collateral blood flow or through treatment in a patient with aphasia and a striatocapsular infarct can reverse the aphasia (the patient may present the late vascular syndrome due to the infarct rather than the initial vascular syndrome due to the hypoperfused area [1, 2, 5, 28].

8. Outcome

Using different functional imaging techniques (perfusion computer tomography, diffusion- and perfusion-weighted magnetic resonance imaging, and positron emission tomography), recent studies have indicated characteristics of aphasia (in hyperacute stage), suggested prognosis (in the era of thrombolysis), and observed even the potential new treatments [such as transcranial magnetic stimulation (TMS)] [2].

8.1 Perfusion computer tomography

Measuring cerebral blood flow and volume enables the definition of maps of penumbra (diminution of cerebral blood flow and normal/increase of cerebral blood volume) and infarct (diminution of cerebral blood flow and volume) in the hyperacute stage of ischemic stroke. It has been demonstrated that penumbra dynamics is the major determinant for aphasia evolution. Saving a cerebral area implicated in a specific language function (naming, etc.) clinically improved this modality [2].

8.2 Diffusion- and perfusion-weighted magnetic resonance imaging: the DWI/PWI mismatch region in acute stroke

Functional MRI studies demonstrated that cerebral tissue at risk of infarction (as indicated by the mismatch of PWI and DWI) can survive if recanalization occurs quickly. This represents the major site explaining postischemic recovery, as proved by language task-specific activation adjacent to the infarct lesion within the region certified by the imaging mismatch.

8.3 The networks for residual language function and recovery after stroke

Different studies using positron emission tomography reported that spontaneous recovery of vascular aphasias still occurs with the persistence of the lesion and it takes place by a few distinct mechanisms. The activation appears in some spared left hemisphere language areas, new left hemisphere areas not commonly involved in language processing (pars orbitalis of the inferior frontal gyrus, anterior insula, and middle frontal gyrus), and right hemisphere areas homotopic to control subjects language network. Interestingly, compensation by the right hemisphere respected the aphasia subtype network, the right F3 being recruited when the left F3 was affected [1, 2].

8.4 Prognosis

Usually, vascular aphasias become less severe in the first 3 months after stroke. The spontaneous recovery depends on the severity of the initial aphasia (which has been related to the lesion location and size), but also on general stroke severity, etiology (ischemic and hemorrhagic), time from onset, age, gender, handedness, treatment, motivation and personality, associated disorders, etc. [1, 2, 5].

Nonfluent aphasia can rarely evolve into fluent aphasia, whereas a fluent aphasia never evolves into a nonfluent aphasia [45].

a. Global aphasia may regress to Broca's aphasia (or less frequently to Wernicke's aphasia). Prognosis for global aphasia persisting at 1 month is poor, because only one-third of aphasics communicate satisfactorily at 2 years [2, 13, 46].

b. Broca's aphasia may transform to anomic-plus aphasia. The prognostic for Broca's aphasia is relatively poor, because only 40% of patients regain ability to communicate satisfactorily [2].

c. Transcortical-motor aphasia may transform to anomic-plus aphasia. The prognosis of transcortical-motor aphasia is relatively good, depending on the severity of spontaneous speech diminution and associated executive and memory impairment.

d. Wernicke's aphasia may transform to conduction aphasia. The prognosis is relatively good, as nearly 60% of patients regain ability to communicate satisfactorily (those involving in conduction aphasics) [2].

e. Conduction aphasia has a relatively good prognosis, because 70% of patients regain ability to communicate [2].

f. Transcortical sensory aphasia has a relatively good prognosis, because 60% of patients regain ability to communicate satisfactorily in everyday activities [2].

g. Anomic aphasia has a good prognosis (they have a good ability to communicate) [2, 13, 46].

The outcome of aphasia at 1 year after stroke can be predicted in the first week [45] by stroke subtype, the phonology score (the strongest predictor), age, educational level, and the Barthel Index score. Severe comprehension impairment is reported as a negative factor for stroke recovery, as the aphasic could not understand the rehabilitation tasks. In 2009, Parkinson et al. [47] observed improvement in object and action naming in chronic vascular aphasics. They noted that better recovery was associated with larger lesion in the anterior regions of the brain and absence of lesion in the subcortical regions.

9. Treatment

9.1 Speech therapy

Vascular aphasics may present some spontaneous language amelioration (spontaneous recovery), but speech therapy can significantly contribute to a better aphasia rehabilitation.

A very good language assessment is the key point for any program of speech therapy (the role of a dedicated and competent neurologist is very important) [48].

Speech therapy should not be used in the hyperacute stage of stroke. In this stage, we should focus on reperfusion (i.v. thrombolysis/thrombectomy) of the affected arterial territory. Speech and language therapy should be typically started as soon as the clinical condition becomes favorable, which is nowadays generally possible in acute stroke units (in the acute/subacute stage of stroke) [2].

The speech therapy has five objectives:

a. *To keep the aphasic verbally active*: the specialists, including the neurologists, speech therapists, psychologists, nurses, and the family have to communicate with the patient using verbal and written language, not only gesture.

b. *To relearn language*: even if the patient is old or present a large infarct, it is generally accepted that he can still relearn some language, from the simpler to the more complex (including the vocabulary or the grammar).

c. *To provide strategies to improve language*: different language abilities can ameliorate if only selective strategies are used (depending on the peculiar type of aphasia; for example, the melodic intonation therapy is efficient only in Broca's aphasias, not in Wernicke's aphasia.

d. *To teach the family to improve communication*: to avoid especially verbal interference, to keep the conversational subject, to use plenty of redundant information, to speak slow, to use prosody, and to be aware that the aphasic's communication ability certainly fluctuates due to variations in attention, etc.

e. *To offer psychological support*: due to his/her communication difficulties, the aphasic needs somebody (the therapist) capable of understanding and supporting him [49].

Bhogal et al. [50] reviewed 10 studies and noted that intense speech therapy over a short period (approximately 9 hours of therapy per week during 12 weeks) ameliorate outcome. Conversely, lower intensity (2 hours a week) over a longer period (more than 20 weeks) did not improve evolution compared with informal support. In conclusion, speech therapy intensity should be of at least of 1 hour per day in the first 3 months after stroke onset [2].

Due to the specific level of the language which is affected, the speech therapy strategy to be used will be different (auditory analysis, word identification, etc.). For example, in global aphasia, the main goals of therapy are represented by helping the patient to use remaining abilities, to restore language abilities, to learn other methods (nonverbal) of communicating, etc. [48].

9.2 Pharmacotherapy

Nowadays, treatment of reperfusion (designed to restore cortical perfusion (i.v. thrombolysis/thrombectomy)) during the first 4–5 h (thrombolysis), and 6–12 h (thrombectomy) from the clinical onset, represents the main prevention approach.

Preliminary positive results were found using piracetam in nonfluent aphasias [51], but it has not been proven to be effective in long-term use [52]. Despite positive preliminary reports, bromocriptine did not improve nonfluent aphasias in a randomized, double-blind, placebo-controlled clinical trial [53]. Preliminary positive results were also noted using cholinergic agents (donepezil) in fluent aphasias [2, 54]. Efficacy of pharmacological treatments in the chronic phase needs to be demonstrated.

9.3 Transcranial magnetic stimulation (TMS)

Functional imaging studies of language in nonfluent aphasics usually report a possible overactivation in right hemisphere language homologues [55].

Evidence exists that left hemisphere functional recovery is clinically more relevant than right hemisphere activation as a compensatory mechanism after stroke. Thus, right hemisphere activation might be a negative factor for aphasia recovery after stroke [55]. Use of TMS could provide right hemisphere inhibition and, therefore, ameliorate regression of language deficits. Preliminary reports suggested that

TMS can improve naming in nonfluent vascular aphasics [55]. This assertion needs to be confirmed by randomized controlled trials.

As a general rule, pharmacological treatment or TMS would be better delivered just before speech and language therapy [2].

10. Conclusions

Vascular aphasia is a term that covers complex syndromes, and it is considered not only a stroke severity marker outcome (it is associated with a higher risk of mortality) but also a poststroke poor functional outcome (can have a dramatic impact on person's ability to communicate and increased risk of developing post-stroke dementia). Taking into consideration the unpredictable evolution of all mentioned aphasic syndromes and the lack of treatment strategies, next researches should focus on combined methods of improving patients' language after acute and even chronic stage of stroke (such as transcranial magnetic stimulation and speech therapy applied in consecutive, consequent, and sustained sessions).

Author details

Dragoş Cătălin Jianu[1,2*], Silviana Nina Jianu[3], Ligia Petrica[4], Traian Flavius Dan[1,2] and Georgiana Munteanu[2]

1 Department of Neurology, "Victor Babes" University of Medicine and Pharmacy, Timisoara, Romania

2 Head of the First Department of Neurology, "Pius Brânzeu" County Emergency Clinical Hospita, Timisoara, Romania

3 Department of Ophthalmology, Military Emergency Hospital, Timisoara, Romania

4 Department of Nephrology, "Victor Babes" University of Medicine and Pharmacy, Timisoara, Romania

*Address all correspondence to: dcjianu@yahoo.com

References

[1] Abou Zeki D, Hillis A. Chapter 12. Acquired disorders of language and speech. In: Masud H, Schott JM, editors. Oxford Textbook of Cognitive Neurology and Dementia. UK: Oxford University Press; 2016. pp. 123-133

[2] Croquelois A, Godefroy O. Chapter 7. Vascular aphasias. In: Godefroy O, editor. The Behavioral and Cognitive Neurology of Stroke. 2nd ed. UK: Cambridge University Press; 2013. pp. 65-75

[3] Alajouanine T. L'aphasie et le langage pathologique. Paris : J.B. Baillière et fils éditeurs; 1968. p. 19

[4] Benson FD, Geschwind N. Chapter 5. Aphasia and related disorders, a clinical approach. In: Principles of Behavioral Neurology. 1989

[5] Jianu DC. Elemente de afaziologie (Romanian). Timisoara, Romania: Mirton; 2001

[6] Ardila A. Chapter 10. Assessment of aphasia. In: Aphasia Handbook 2. Miami, Florida, USA: Florida International University; 2014. pp. 171-188

[7] De Renzi E, Faglioni P. Normative data and screening power of a shortened version of the token test. Cortex. 1978;7:41-49

[8] Goodglass H, Kaplan E, editors. The Assessment of Aphasia and Related Disorders. 2nd ed. Philadelphia, PA: Lea and Febiger; 1983

[9] Kertesz A. The Western Aphasia Battery. New York: Grune & Stratton; 1982

[10] Nespoulous JL, Lecours AR, Lafond D, editors. Protocole Montreal—Toulouse de l'examen de l'aphasie: Module Standard Initial (Version Beta). Montreal: L'Ortho Edition; 1986

[11] Kertesz A, Sheppard A. The epidemiology of aphasic and cognitive impairment in stroke: Age, sex, aphasia type an laterality differences. Brain. 1981;**104**:117-128

[12] Nadeau SE, Crosson B. Subcortical aphasia. Brain and Language. 1997;**58**:355-402

[13] Verstichel P. Thalamic aphasia. Revue Neurologique (Paris). 2003;**122**:947-957

[14] Lhermitte F, Derouesné J. L'aphasie amnéstique. Revue Neurologique. 1976;**132**:669-685

[15] Kearns KP. Chapter 8. Broca's aphasia. In: La Pointe LL, editor. Aphasia and Related Neurogenic Language Disorders. 3rd ed. New York, Stuttgart: Thieme; 2005. pp. 117-141

[16] Alexander MP, Naeser MA. Broca's area aphasics. Brain and Language. 1992;**43**(3):215-227

[17] Haartmann HJ, Kolk HHJ. The production of grammatical morphology in Broca's and Wernicke's aphasics. Cortex. 1992;**28**:97-112

[18] Jianu DC, Bednar M, Zolog A. Diagnosticul diferențial între tulburările fonetice şi fonologice la afazici (Romanian). Neurologie, Psihiatrie, Psihologie, Psihoterapie. (Revista Societății de Neurologie şi Psihiatrie pentru Copii şi adolescenți din România), Bucuresti, Romania. 1999;**2**:55-58

[19] Jianu DC. Managementul afazicilor romani consecutiv infarctelor cerebrale (Romanian). Timisoara, Romania: Mirton; 2011

[20] Damasio AR. Aphasia. New England Journal of Medicine. 1992;**326**:531-539

[21] Kertesz A. Clinical forms of aphasia. Acta Neurochirurgica. Supplementum (Wien). 1993;**56**:52-58

[22] Kory Calomfirescu S, Kory Mercea M. Afazia în accidentele vasculare cerebrale (Romanian). Cluj-Napoca, Romania: Casa Cărţii de Ştiinţă; 1996

[23] Thompson CK. Chapter 2. Functional neuroimaging. In: La Pointe LL, editor. Aphasia and Related Neurogenic Language Disorders. 3rd ed. New York-Stuttgart: Thieme; 2005. pp. 19-38

[24] Hanna D. Chapter I. Neuroimaging contributions to the understanding of aphasia. In: Boller F, editor. Handbook of Neuropsychology. Vol. 2. Amsterdam, Netherlands: Elsevier Science Publishers, B.V.; 1989

[25] Poeck K, de Bleser R, von Keyserlink DG. Computed tomography localization of standard aphasic syndromes. In: Rose FC, editor. Advances in Neurology. Vol. 42: Progress in Aphasiology. New York: Raven Press; 1984. pp. 71-89

[26] Caspari I. Chapter 9. Wernicke's aphasia. In: La Pointe LL, editor. Aphasia and Related Neurogenic Language Disorders. 3rd ed. New York-Stuttgart: Thieme; 2005. pp. 142-154

[27] Gainotti G, Ibba A, Caltagirone C. Perturbations acoustiques et semantiques de la compréhension dans l'aphasie. Revue Neurologique (Paris). 1975;**131**(9):645-659

[28] Jianu DC, Petrica M, Matcău L, Zolog A. Observaţii anatomo-clinice asupra unor cazuri de afazie fluentă Wernicke (Romanian). Neurologia Medico-Chirurgica. 2001;**6**(1):69-79

[29] Simmons-Mackie N. Chapter 10. Conduction aphasia. In: La Pointe LL, editor. Aphasia and Related Neurogenic Language Disorders. 3rd ed. New York-Stuttgart: Thieme; 2005. pp. 155-168

[30] Benson FD, Sheremata WA, Bouchard R, et al. Conduction aphasia, a clinico-pathological study. Archives of Neurology. 1973;**38**:339-346

[31] Geschwind N. Disconnection syndromes in animals and man: Part 1. Brain. 1965;**88**:237-294

[32] Jianu DC. Observaţii asupra unui caz de afazie de conducţie (Romanian). Neurologia Medico-Chirurgica. 1996;**1**(1):35-38

[33] Cimino-Knight A, Hollingsworth AL, Gonzalez Rothi LJ. Chapter 11. The transcortical aphasias. In: La Pointe LL, editor. Aphasia and Related Neurogenic Language Disorders. 3rd ed. New York-Stuttgart: Thieme; 2005. pp. 169-185

[34] Jianu DC. Observaţii asupra unui caz de afazie paroxistică prin interesarea ariei motorii suplimentare Penfield, în cursul evoluţiei unui meningiom de sinus longitudinal superior (Romanian). Neurologia Medico-Chirurgica. 1998;**5**(2):51-53

[35] Jianu DC, Petrica M, Deme S, Scutelnicu D, Matcău L, Zolog A, et al. Consideraţii anatomo-clinice asupra unor cazuri de afazie transcorticală motorie, senzorială şi mixtă (Romanian). Neurologia Medico-Chirurgica. 2000;**5**(1):45-54

[36] Grossi D et al. Mixed transcortical aphasia: Clinical features and neuroanatomical corelates. European Neurology. 1991;**31**:204-211

[37] Collins M. Chapter 12. Global aphasia. In: La Pointe LL, editor. Aphasia and Related Neurogenic Language Disorders. 3rd ed. New York-Stuttgart: Thieme; 2005. pp. 186-198

[38] Hanlon RE, Lux WE, Dromerick AW. Global aphasia without hemiparesis: Language profiles and lesion distribution. Journal

of Neurology, Neurosurgery, and Psychiatry (England). 1999;**66**(3):365-369

[39] Godefroy O, Dubois C, Debachy B, Leclerc M, Kreisler A. Vascular aphasias: Main characteristics of patients hospitalized in acute stroke units. Stroke. 2002;**33**:702-705

[40] Oldfield RC. The assessment and analysis of handedness: The Edinburgh inventory. Neuropsychologia. 1971;**9**:97-113

[41] LaPointe LL. Aphasia and Related Neurogenic Language Disorders. 3rd ed. Tallahassee, Florida: Department of Communication Disorders, Florida State University; 2005

[42] Kreisler A, Godefroy O, Delmaire C, et al. The anatomy of aphasia revisited. Neurology. 2000;**54**(5):1117-1123

[43] Coppens P. Why are Wernicke's aphasia patients older than Broca's? A critical view of the hypotheses. Aphasiology. 1991;**5**:279-290

[44] Lecours AR, Lhermitte F, Bryans B. Aphasiology. London: Baillière-Tindall; 1983

[45] El Hachioui H, Lingsma HF, van de Sandt-Koenderman MWME, Dippel DWJ, Koudstall PJ, Visch-Brink EG. Long term prognosis of aphasia after stroke. Journal of Neurology, Neurosurgery, and Psychiatry. 2013;**84**:310-315

[46] Jianu DC, Jianu SN, Dan TF, Munteanu G. Extra and transcranial color-coded sonography findings in aphasics with internal carotid artery, and/or left middle cerebral artery stenosis or occlusion. European Journal of Neurology. 2018;**25**(Suppl 1):35-36

[47] Parkinson BR, Raymer A, Chang YL, Fitzgerald DB, Crosson B. Lesion characteristics related to treatment improvement in object and action naming for patients with chronic aphasia. Brain and Language. 2009;**40**:23-23

[48] Ardila A. Chapter 12. Aphasia rehabilitation. In: Aphasia Handbook 2. Miami, Florida, USA: Florida International University; 2014. pp. 198-208

[49] Ardila A. Chapter 11. Recovery and prognosis in aphasia. In: Aphasia Handbook 2. Miami, Florida, USA: Florida International University; 2014. pp. 189-197

[50] Bhogal SK, Teasell R, Speechley M. Intensity of aphasia therapy, impact on recovery. Stroke. 2003;**34**:987-993

[51] Greener J, Enderby P, Whurr R. Speech and language therapy for aphasia following stroke. Cochrane Database of Systematic Reviews. 2001;**2**:CD000125

[52] Güngör L, Terzi M, Onar MK. Does long term use of piracetam improve speech disturbances due to ischemic cerebrovascular diseases? Brain and Language, Elsevier. 2011;**117**:23-27

[53] Ashtary F, Janghorhani M, Chitsaz A, Reisi M, Bahrami A. A randomized, double-blind trial of bromocriptine efficacy in nonfluent aphasia after stroke. Neurology. 2006;**27**:97-98

[54] Berthier ML. Poststroke aphasia: Epidemiology, pathophysiology and treatment. Drugs & Aging. 2005;**22**:163-182

[55] Naeser MA, Martin PI, Ho M, et al. Transcranial magnetic stimulation and aphasia rehabilitation. Archives of Physical Medicine and Rehabilitation. 2012;**93**:S26-S34

Chapter 4

Telestroke: A New Paradigm

Rohan Sharma, Krishna Nalleballe, Nidhi Kapoor, Vasuki Dandu, Karthika Veerapaneni, Sisira Yadala, Madhu Jasti, Suman Siddamreddy, Sanjeeva Onteddu and Aliza Brown

Abstract

Stroke is one of the leading causes of death and disability across the world. With the development of new modalities of treatment, including the use of intravenous tissue plasminogen activator and mechanical thrombectomy, clinical outcomes have improved in patients with acute ischemic strokes. However, these interventions are time dependent, and there exists a great disparity between the rural and urban parts of the world in terms of the availability of neurologists and these lifesaving treatment options. Telestroke networks utilize digital technology for two-way, high-resolution video teleconferencing to help abate these disparities by bringing safe, efficient, and cost-effective care to underserved communities in the United States and around the world.

Keywords: telestroke, acute ischemic stroke, tPA, teleconference, quality measures

1. Introduction

In the United States (US), stroke is the fifth leading cause of mortality with a stroke occurring approximately every 40 seconds and stroke-related death approximately every 4 minutes [1, 2]. In 2011, stroke was found to be the leading cause of disability in the US, with around 7 million stroke survivors [3]. In 2016, the World Health Organization designated stroke as the second leading cause of mortality worldwide. Acute ischemic strokes account for about 80% of all stroke-related deaths [4]. Intravenous tissue plasminogen activator (tPA) has been shown to improve outcomes in acute ischemic stroke [5, 6]. In patients who receive tPA, early administration has been shown to reduce morbidity, mortality, and adverse events such as intracranial hemorrhages, promoting early discharges and higher rates of independent ambulation at discharge [5, 7]. Mechanical thrombectomies performed by neuro-interventionists have shown to improve outcomes for patients with proximal intracranial arterial occlusion [8–11] and have become the standard of care for patients who qualify for intervention. However, this procedure is performed only at tertiary care centers and is not available at smaller hospitals around the country.

Despite the obvious benefits of tPA administration, only a small percentage of patients presenting with acute ischemic strokes are eligible to receive it [12–15]. The most common reason attributed to this is a delay between the development of stroke symptoms and the patient seeking treatment at a hospital [16, 17]. There are also marked rural–urban disparities in stroke care [18–20]. These disparities are, in part, a result of the scarcity of neurologists [21–24]. Studies have shown better outcomes in stroke patients under the care of neurologists as compared to physicians of other specialties, such as Internal Medicine or Family Medicine [22, 25, 26]. Telestroke aims to bridge this gap by providing neurology expertise in remote areas around the world through high-quality audio-video conferencing and digital image sharing.

2. Historical perspective

Communication of medical information across long distances has occurred throughout history. It is well documented that bonfires and heliographs were used to send communications about the bubonic plague in Europe [27]. Telegraph communication was used in the civil war and radio communication was used in World War I, and wars thereafter, to send information about casualties and to request medical dispatches and transport for wounded soldiers [28]. Telemedicine in its current form was developed by NASA to monitor the physiologic states of astronauts during manned space missions [29]. The first interactive video telemedicine systems were established for psychiatry [30] and radiology [31] but later expanded to critical care [32] and oncology [33] to bridge the shortage of specialists in these fields. In 1999, the term *telestroke* was first coined by Levine and Gorman, who described the use of video telecommunications as a means to facilitate cerebrovascular consults to remote areas adding great expertise to the care of stroke patients [34]. Since then the number of telestroke networks around the world has expanded significantly [35–38].

3. Telestroke models

Before discussing telestroke models, it is important to understand the terminology used to describe telestroke systems, as described by the American Telemedicine Association [39].

1. Distant site: the distant telestroke provider location.

2. Originating site: the site where the patient is initially located.

3. Telestroke network: a group of primary, secondary, and tertiary care settings that provide acute stroke care to patient populations. Telestroke networks consist of originating sites where the patients are located and distant sites where the telestroke provider is located.

4. Spoke: the affiliate or partner site in a telestroke network that is underserviced or under-supported by neurologists where patient services are delivered.

5. Hub: a comprehensive tertiary care center where vascular neurologists and other acute stroke specialists compose a call panel delivering telestroke services to network partner sites (i.e., spoke sites). This is also the center where the patient may be transferred if a higher level of care is needed.

Several different telestroke models have been described and are listed below [38, 39].

1. Hub and spoke within a single healthcare system.

2. Hub and spoke with external sites.

3. Horizontal hubless network: interconnected sites within a large hospital system for on-call clinical coverage.

4. Third-party distribution model: telestroke services are provided to multiple originating sites through arrangements with an independent corporation or an affiliated network of telestroke providers.

5. Supervisory training model: academic teleneurology programs to assist trainees within the hospital system.

Hub and Spoke with external sites and third-party distribution models are the most commonly used models within telestroke [35]. In telestroke networks, the majority of spoke sites are small hospitals (i.e., 0–99 beds) [37], but the spoke hospital size may vary from 25 to 500 beds in different telestroke networks [17]. A telestroke consult typically starts with a patient presenting to a spoke site with a suspected stroke. After an initial assessment by the physician at the spoke site, a triage process is conducted through telephone operators, followed by a video teleconferencing call with the neurologist at the distant site [see flow diagram of a telestroke system]. After reviewing the National Institute of Health Stroke Scale (NIHSS) and brain imaging (typically a non-contrasted CT scan of the head) and reviewing the patient's history for indications/contraindications for tPA, a decision is made for administration of tPA. After this initial process, the decision of transferring the patient to the hub site is made, depending upon the need for further investigation, possible thrombectomy/neurosurgical intervention, or requirement of a higher level of care as compared to the spoke site. The term "Drip and Ship" is often used to describe transfer from spoke to hub sites, where after receiving the bolus dose of tPA, the patient is started on tPA drip and transferred emergently for further management [40].

The majority of the hospitals in telestroke systems have formal written contracts between the hub and the spoke site with a closed-loop communication system in place [37]. A vast array of Food and Drug Administration (FDA) approved two-way video-conferencing modalities with picture archiving and communication system are available for use by these networks that provide Health Insurance Portability and Accountability Act (HIPPA) compliant, secure, encrypted multipoint data sharing with evolving functionality through the use of desktops, robotic carts, laptops, tablets, and even mobile phones with provider-to-provider interfaces [37, 38].

More recent advancements in telestroke systems include an ambulance-based telemedicine system that provides a feasible tool for prehospital stroke assessment [41–44]. Early attempts at prehospital telestroke consults were limited due to technical difficulties [44]. Newer studies have shown a high level of agreement in evaluation and treatment by mobile stroke units with a vascular neurologist on board compared to telestroke consults by a vascular neurologist [45] at a distant site who guides immediate treatment [46]. The data, however, is still limited and requires further investigation before the utility and efficacy of telestroke programs can be ascertained.

4. Effectiveness and utility of telestroke in management of acute ischemic stroke

The primary goal of telestroke models is to establish a network of neurology consults across underserved areas that do not have in-house neurology consultants available, thereby expediting the initial stroke exam and care. As the effective tPA window is time-sensitive, and early administration of tPA is known to improve outcomes [5, 6, 13, 47], delay in transport of patients to tertiary care centers can lead to loss of the crucial intervention time window in acute ischemic stroke patients. After adequate training, the use of telestroke systems to measure NIHSS scores is viable and scoring is reliable, with inter-rater reliability comparable to that of in-person measurements [48, 49] even in telemedicine-naïve stroke practitioners [50]. Such assessment has also been found to be reliable when performed by neurology trained nurse practitioners [51], on laptop-based workstations [52], or even mobile-based video telestroke consults [53, 54]. Also, the FDA has approved teleradiology systems that enable effective and rapid evaluation of images by stroke specialists [55]. Stroke specialist evaluation via teleradiology systems has been found to be comparable to assessment by a neuroradiologist in aiding the decision making for tPA administration [56, 57].

Studies have shown that telestroke facilitated administration of tPA to patients in community hospitals and rural hospitals (as small as 100 beds or less) has outcomes comparable to those of in-person treatment at comprehensive stroke care centers [58–61]. Even with in a stroke network, the performance of spoke sites is similar regardless of the bedsize [62]. Also, the use of telestroke at rural hospitals can provide patients with comparable or reduced time between symptom onset and tPA administration [door-to-needle time (DTN)] compared to those directly presenting to tertiary care centers [63]. A non-blinded randomized control trial in the Telemedic Pilot Project for Integrative Stroke Care (TEMPiS) network in Germany showed that patients treated in telestroke network hospitals had significantly fewer poor outcomes compared to patients treated in community hospitals without telestroke capabilities [64]. Telestroke consults are becoming exceedingly cost-effective in dealing with acute strokes in the community [65–69].

5. Telestroke for post-tPA care and work up

Telestroke consults also have utility beyond acute stroke. Patients receiving tPA or those with subacute strokes with milder symptoms not requiring emergent intravascular intervention can remain at the spoke site for further investigation. Telestroke follow-up consults can aid in guiding the physicians at the spoke sites to continue further stroke workup and discharge patients from the spoke site. This may also reduce the cost of transport and limit patients being transferred to hub sites to only those requiring urgent neurosurgical/intravascular intervention. A randomized control trial by Evans et al. showed that the management of stroke patients in dedicated stroke units showed better outcomes for large vessel infarcts but not for small lacunar infarcts when compared to those in general medical wards with stroke team support [70]. Based on this hypothesis, small lacunar strokes could potentially be managed by the medical team at spokes sites with telestroke consults and follow-ups. The Telemedicine in Stroke in Swabia Project and The Order of St. Francis Stroke Network study experience demonstrated the safety and reliability of such telestroke models [71, 72]. Even for patients requiring treatment in an intensive care unit, teleneurointensive care units are providing valuable support for prevention, diagnosis, and the timely management of cerebrovascular conditions induced secondary to neurologic injuries [73] and have shown improved outcomes [74].

Telestroke has also been studied in in-home and ambulatory post-stroke rehabilitation settings for serial neurologic assessments and timely adjustments of therapies. These studies have shown that telerehabilitation approaches are comparable to conventional rehabilitation in improving activities of daily living and motor function for stroke survivors [75, 76]. Virtual neurovascular clinics aimed at secondary stroke prevention are another evolving avenue for follow-up visits for stroke patients [77].

In the field of clinical research, telestroke consults may aid in identifying patients who are eligible for trials of therapies for ischemic or hemorrhagic strokes, neuroprotective agents, or innovative diagnostic tests, thereby facilitating expedited enrollment at the originating sites after transfer to stroke centers [78]. Telestroke models are being incorporated into the education and training of neurologists, emergency teams, and nursing staff [77, 79–82]. With the ever-expanding horizons of telestroke, training in telemedicine will likely become mainstream for all future physician and medical personnel training programs. However, the data regarding the use of telestroke beyond acute stroke care is still limited and needs further investigation.

6. Telestroke outcomes and cost-effectiveness

Zaidi et al. showed that outcomes at 90 days were no different between patients treated with tPA by telemedicine and patients treated by the same neurologists over the same time interval at the stroke center hub hospital [83]. They also found no difference in time from stroke onset to treatment. Switzer et al. found that the average time between symptom onset and treatment at the spoke sites in their telestroke system was lower than the emergency department at their hub site [63]. As previously mentioned, several studies have found post-tPA outcomes at spoke sites were comparable to those of in-person treatment at comprehensive stroke care centers [58–61]. Implementation of a standardized regional telestroke program in a community setting increased utilization of alteplase, improved DTN time, decreased length of stay, and significantly increased the chances of patients going home [84].

Establishing a telestroke network requires infrastructure and technology-related expenses along with the expenses of round-the-clock neurology coverage and the cost of transport. Initial projects around the country were supported by government funds and research grants, but to develop a self-sustaining model, telestroke networks need to be cost-effective. For a Danish telestroke system consisting of five hubs and five spokes, a 2008 study by Ehlers et al. calculated an incremental cost-effectiveness ratio (the cost of thrombolysis per quality-adjusted life year [QALY]) to be approximately US$50,000 after 1 year [69]. In 2011, Nelson et al. conducted cost data analyses of telestroke networks in rural Arizona and Utah and found the incremental cost-effectiveness ratio using a 90-day horizon of $108,363 per QALY and a lifetime horizon of $2449 per QALY [66], which reflected a high initial cost but overall long-term cost reduction, likely due to rehabilitation cost reduction from early tPA administration. Also, the highest cost-effectiveness was seen in the most severe stroke cases. In a 2013 study by Switzer et al., cost savings of $358,435 per year over 5 years were observed in a telestroke system consisting of one hub and seven spokes, as well as an improvement in patients' quality of life associated with increased numbers of individuals being discharged to home [67]. Growing evidence for the cost-effectiveness of telestroke networks and improved patient outcomes has spurred the growth of telestroke networks around the world.

7. Telestroke quality measures

Continuous quality improvement is a key element for any successful telestroke program. Several elements play a role in this improvement, including adaptation to local laws and statues, effective training programs, identification of competency issues, and overcoming challenges with technical and manpower issues at both provider and recipient sites. In 1988, Donebedian was the first to describe the model of structure, process, and outcomes measurements for assessing the quality of healthcare [85]. Systematic collection and analysis of quality data has been shown to improve the quality of stroke care that is delivered [86], and telestroke is no exception to this. Several quality measures help assess and quantify the overall function of telestroke systems. Most hub hospitals have stroke certification and emergency and ICU staff training through standards set by the Joint Commission on the Accreditation of Healthcare Organizations (JCAHO) process.

7.1 Structural measures

The capacity of the healthcare system, staffing ratios of specialists, availability of specialized units and equipment, and the organization structure with hospital networking should all be carefully studied and analyzed for any telehealth network systems. Defined protocols should be in place both at the originating and distant sites.

7.2 Process measures

Analogous to the traditional stroke pathway, the key global component of telestroke quality is still DTN time. Median DTN with telestroke varies from 106 to 121 minutes, even though the recommendation is less than 1 hour [58]. Several aspects of stroke chain-of-care that play an important role in DTN include Emergency Department (ED) door to CT scan (D-CT) time, ED door to tele-neurologist consult time, teleneurologist to camera/phone time, and teleconsult duration (Con).

Clear definitions of these times are important as no uniform definitions currently exist. In some centers, a consult with teleneurologist occurs after CT scan results are obtained, while in other centers, a consult is initiated even before the CT scan is ordered. The time from ED to consult differs in these situations, which can affect these measures. Similarly, the definition of consult time varies between centers. At some centers, consult time is defined as the time spent on camera evaluating patients, and at other centers, it is defined as time spent on camera along with the time spent reviewing the images and other diagnostic results. Because of these variations, consult duration varied from 14 to 32 minutes in different studies [87, 88]. Studies showed that telestroke by itself might not decrease the DTN as there are variations in the subsects of stroke chain-of-care [89].

It has been shown that D-NC and Con play a major role in DTN [90]. Various factors including, when the consultant is notified, the time a consultant takes to interview the patient, and the experience level of the staff aiding with the examination will have to be considered while analyzing such data. The percentage of patients transferred after a telestroke consult to a destination hospital is also an important factor as it involves significant costs [67]. Data should be collected quantifying the rate of transfers after the consult and steps should be taken to minimize unnecessary transfers.

7.3 Outcome measures

The success of any program is ultimately decided by measuring outcomes, which could be patient related or system related. A modified Rankin scale, which is measured 90 days after a stroke, is the most commonly used measurement of stroke outcome [83]. Steps should be taken to ensure a 90-day follow-up on all the telestroke treated patients. No significant differences in mortality or morbidity were noted in patients in the hub and spoke hospitals of the TEMPiS network [91]. Even though 90-day outcomes after stroke are reported in most clinical trials, this data is not routinely collected by hospitals because of the cost and complexity involved. Data on stroke mimics that were treated by telestroke networks is an important factor as it plays a big role in minimizing costs, even though tPA administration might not increase the risk to these patients. Similarly, data on the percentage of patients receiving tPA through telestroke networks is very useful to compare with in-person stroke treatment numbers. In a study that examined several telestroke networks, the rate of tPA via telestroke was 18–36% compared to the national average tPA administration rate of 5–8% [91].

7.4 Patient/provider-related outcomes

Data collection regarding patient characteristics, NIHSS score pre/post-treatment and before discharge, length of hospital stay, discharge disposition (home vs. rehab vs. sub-acute rehab), readmission rate, complications including intracranial hemorrhage, other significant hemorrhages, mortality, and 90-day follow-up outcomes are recommended by the American Heart Association and the American Stroke Association [92]. One of the highest priorities for several healthcare systems is patient satisfaction. Attempts should be made to follow-up with the treated patients and family members about their satisfaction with the telestroke process. LaMonte et al. found that the telestroke process enhanced patient satisfaction in their study [93]. Measuring provider satisfaction is equally important for improving telestroke service quality. Studies showed that patients are more enthusiastic about telemedicine compared to providers even though both of the groups were satisfied [94]. Providers having less of a personal benefit was one of the possible reasons behind this discrepancy [92].

7.5 Technological quality measures

In a good telestroke program, the technology involved is as important as the physicians' clinical expertise. Video and audio conferencing equipment quality, transmission clarity, internet speed, user-friendliness of the software, accessibility of personnel training modules, and encryption of patient information in transit to protect patient privacy all play a role for effective delivery of telestroke care. All technical difficulties, failures, and limitations should be continuously monitored, documented, and analyzed promptly to prevent repeated occurrences.

Lastly, apart from the issues unique to telestroke, data on regular measures as recommended by National Quality Forum for stroke patients, including use of tPA, anti-thrombolysis therapy by day 2, thromboembolism prophylaxis, lipid-lowering medications on discharge, anti-thrombotic therapy on discharge, anticoagulation in the setting of atrial fibrillation, rehabilitation evaluation, and stroke education should be collected and evaluated regularly [95].

7.6 Quality measures: final thoughts

There are still challenges with current models. In the last 15 years, there has been a substantial improvement in stroke quality measures. Most of the measures are already being performed with a high compliance rate and innovation. They should be expanded to pre-hospitalization and post-hospitalization settings as well as to telestroke for further improvement of stroke care [62, 96–99]. Universal guidelines about definitions of times in stroke chain-of-care, protocols for consultant notification, and specific standard stepwise processes that can be applied universally for telestroke networks will be useful in standardizing telestroke models. As telestroke is becoming more popular in delivering care for acute stroke patients, there is a need for strict quality metrics to ensure safe and effective care for the patients. Even though in several aspects telestroke is as effective as in-person stroke care, there are several issues pertinent to telestroke like technology, policies, and challenges with data collection due to distant participating sites that need to be refined for effective and timely management of stroke patients.

8. Telestroke across the world

Lack of neurology coverage is not unique to the US; it is a problem worldwide [100]. Several countries in Europe have developed efficient telestroke networks [59, 64, 69, 101–103], with the TEMPiS network in Germany showing remarkable results [64, 104, 105]. The Telestroke Committee of the European Stroke Organization has recently published recommendations regarding telestroke networks in Europe concerning infrastructure, teleconsultation service, transfer options, standard operating procedures, professional training, and quality monitoring and improvement. They have also made recommendations about the technical and ethical aspects of telemedicine [106], which are similar to ones in the US.

Asia is quite heterogeneous in terms of variability in language, governments, culture, historical links, socioeconomic development, and organization of health services. In China, the National Telestroke Center, established in 2014, was designed to provide neurological coverage to 300 rural hospitals throughout the country through the telestroke network [107]. This was also the first platform where Google Glasses were used for real-time telestroke consults. The system is still evolving and data from China is still limited. In India, telestroke systems are still uncommon, but they show prospects for expansion, aiming to provide care to rural communities that are limited in their resources [108, 109]. Japan, Singapore, and South Korea have rather advanced nationwide medical systems, but telemedicine experience in these countries is still limited [110–112]. Teleneurology and telestroke have great potential to extend neurology expertise to underserved populations in the world; however, further investment in creating infrastructure and technology is needed before their impact on healthcare is realized.

9. Telestroke in the new era of novel coronavirus (COVID-19)

In December 2019, the first case of the novel coronavirus COVID-19 was identified in China [113]. Since then, the rapid spread of the virus has led to a worldwide pandemic [114]. The US has become the epicenter of this pandemic with the largest number of reported cases worldwide. Of all COVID-19 cases, an estimated 19% are healthcare personnel [115]. The COVID-19 pandemic has put a significant strain on healthcare personnel in providing in-person care, especially in an acute setting. Several States in the US and countries around the world have implemented stay-at-home orders. Hospitals have canceled elective procedures and outpatient in-person clinic visits to minimize the exposure risk to patients and healthcare workers. Additionally, COVID-19 is associated with an increased risk of thromboembolic complications [116]. This puts neurologists at risk of exposure while assessing patients with acute neurological deficits. Screening for symptoms of COVID-19 has also become difficult in the setting of neurological deficits, especially aphasia and encephalopathy. Most countries around the world, including the US, already suffer from a lack of adequate neurology coverage [100] and COVID-19 exposure not only puts neurologists' wellbeing and life at risk but also exacerbates this deficiency. This pandemic has brought the need and utility of telemedicine, teleneurology, and telestroke into the limelight [117–120]. Teleconsults are an effective way of providing outpatient care as well was acute care inside the hospitals, limiting the exposure risk to physicians and patients, as well as limiting the use of personal protective equipment which is in short supply. The pandemic may change the paradigm of teleneurology and telestroke permanently and force the system to adapt to its growing need at a much faster pace.

10. Hurdles and barriers

Despite the utility and efficacy of telestroke networks, there exist significant hurdles in establishing and efficiently sustaining a viable telestroke program.

10.1 Issues regarding reimbursement

The most important hurdle is third party reimbursement. It took decades for the concept of telemedicine to come to fruition, and pay parity kept telemedicine programs across the country from flourishing, sustaining, and expanding [121–126]. Without appropriate reimbursement, the burden of financial overhead in maintaining the high-quality video interface, teleneurology and teleradiology coverage, and costs of emergent care including imaging, tPA, and transportation to hub hospitals would make telestroke network unsustainable. The Centers for Medicare and Medicaid Services (CMS) has addressed the need for reimbursement for telemedicine services and third-party payers have followed suit [37, 121]. Appropriate reimbursement for teleservices remains a concern among providers [127] and continues to be a barrier for the expansion of telestroke networks to underserved areas of the country.

10.2 Licensure and credentialing constraints

Licensure and hospital credentialing, often across state lines, further burdens physicians and hospitals to spend resources, thus putting additional constraints on the expansion of these services. Physicians are required to maintain a license in the state where the spoke site is located in addition to the hub site where they usually work. This requires unrestricted licensure to be maintained in every state where the teleconsult is requested. A national or multistate license for telemedicine would reduce the necessity for a consultant to be licensed in multiple individual states, but this kind of license does not currently exist [128]. In 2011, CMS began allowing credentialing and privileging by proxy at small and critical-access hospitals, which has allowed these hospitals to rely on the credentialing and privileging process performed at the hub site [92, 129]. However, this policy needs to be adopted by all 50 states to mitigate the onus of licensing and credentialing on physicians and small hospitals. Also, reimbursement in cases where the patient receives tPA at the spoke site and is transferred to the hub hospital remains an issue, as neither the spoke nor hub facility is eligible to bill the higher Medicare diagnosis-related group codes that are associated with thrombolytic administration [128].

10.3 Infrastructure and technological challenges

Establishing and maintaining the infrastructure for high-quality video conferencing in small rural hospitals also adds to the financial burden on these hospitals. There is also marked heterogeneity in the platforms available, which spoke sites need to take into account before joining a telestroke model [37, 128]. Platform differences also limit the flexibility of these rural hospitals in terms of associating with more than one network or transitioning to a different network as the platforms utilized by these networks may be incompatible. Additionally, to comply with CMS billing requirements, a high-quality, two-way video connection is recommended and a minimum frame rate of at least 20 frames per second has been suggested [130]. Thus, high-speed internet is an essential component of telestroke networks. The availability of high-speed internet connections in rural parts of the country is limited and is a separate problem limiting the implementation of telestroke networks. These issues become exceedingly challenging in resource-limited countries around the world.

10.4 Physician buy-in and telestroke staff training

Convincing the leadership of potential spoke sites of the cost-effectiveness of joining a telestroke system requires time and effort on the part of the hub telestroke providers. Joining a telestroke system not only requires investment in infrastructure but also requires extensive training and development of protocols for teleconsults and transfers. These requirements may appear daunting to the leadership and hospital staff, especially at small rural hospitals with limited resources. However, the literature supporting the safety, cost-effectiveness, and improved patient outcomes related to telestroke networks may help encourage their buy-in to such programs. Joining such a system implies a long-term partnership between the hub and the spoke sites. Trust also needs to be established between the spoke site ED staff and consulting neurologists. Endorsements and testimony from the leadership of existing spoke sites in similar settings, hearing patient experiences from those who benefitted from these networks, and meeting with the team of consulting neurologists may prove useful in building this trust.

Along with the establishment of infrastructure for telestroke, medical staff at spokes sites need to be trained for ever-evolving telestroke protocols and joint commission requirements. They need to be able to recognize the early signs and symptoms of acute stroke, perform NIHSS exams, screen for eligibility for tPA, and to be proficient at using the teleconsult interface to facilitate the process efficiently. Telestroke systems can include stroke patient management training to spoke medical staff on education NIHSS exam demonstrations, reviews of alteplase reconstitution, administration and considerations, alteplase dosage calculations and telemedicine cart demonstration and review. Other patient management training can be provided to paramedics local to the spoke sites, these sessions typically include; impact of and time sensitivity of strokes, what is a stroke, types of stroke, stroke mimics, EMS neurological assessments, stroke management/prehospital guidelines and telemedicine and alteplase through an organizational system of care.

Given the wide variability of telestroke systems based on AHA/ASA guidelines and local governing factors, each network should develop an standard operating protocol (SOP) that suits their needs (**Tables 1–3**) [131]. The volume of teleconsults can vary greatly between the spoke hospitals, thus training needs to be reinforced at specified intervals to ensure efficient and seamless consults and to maintain high-quality patient care. This may lead to telemedicine fatigue in the staff at low-volume hospitals that needs to be mitigated during the training by emphasizing the importance of their work in the teleconsult system in their community at improving

American College of Cardiology/American Heart Association class of recommendation and level of evidence to clinical strategies, interventions, treatments, or diagnostic testing in patient care*
Class (strength) of recommendation
Class I (strong)—benefit >>> risk
Suggested phrases for writing recommendations: • Is recommended • Is indicated/useful/effective/beneficial • Should be performed/administered/others • Comparative-effectiveness phrases†: ○ Treatment/strategy A is recommended/indicated in preference to treatment B ○ Treatment A should be chosen over treatment B
Class IIa (moderate)—benefit >> risk
Suggested phrases for writing recommendations: • Is reasonable • Can be useful/effective/beneficial • Comparative-effectiveness phrases†: ○ Treatment/strategy A is probably recommended/indicated in preference to treatment B ○ It is reasonable to choose treatment A over treatment B
Class IIb (weak)—benefit ≥ risk
Suggested phrases for writing recommendations: • May/might be reasonable • May/might be considered • Usefulness/effectiveness is unknown/unclear/uncertain or not well established
Class III: no benefit (moderate) (generally, LOE A or B use only)—benefit = risk
Suggested phrases for writing recommendations: • Is not recommended • Is not indicated/useful/effective/beneficial • Should not be performed/administered/others
Class III: harm (strong)—risk > benefit
Suggested phrases for writing recommendations: • Potentially harmful • Causes harm • Associated with excess morbidity/mortality • Should not be performed/administered/others

**The outcome or result of the intervention should be specified (an improved clinical outcome or increased diagnostic accuracy or incremental prognostic information).*
†For comparative-effectiveness recommendations (COR I and IIa; LOE A and B only), studies that support the use of comparator verbs should involve direct comparisons of the treatments or strategies being evaluated.

Table 1.
American Heart Association summary of recommendations for telestrokes [131].

outcomes in patients who may have otherwise not had an opportunity for timely stroke intervention due to time lost in transportation to larger centers.

10.5 Data security and sharing

Telestroke networks, like traditional practices, are required to be compliant with HIPAA, which governs protected health information in the US. Given that telestroke

Level A
• High-quality evidence‡ from more than one randomized controlled trial (RCT) • Meta-analyses of high-quality RCTs • One or more RCTs corroborated by high-quality registry studies
Level B-R (randomized)
• Moderate-quality evidence‡ from one or more RCTs • Meta-analyses of moderate-quality RCTs
Level B-NR (nonrandomized)
• Moderate-quality evidence‡ from one or more well-designed, well-executed nonrandomized studies, observational studies, or registry studies • Meta-analyses of such studies
Level C-LD (limited data)
• Randomized or nonrandomized observational or registry studies with limitations of design or execution • Meta-analyses of such studies • Physiological or mechanistic studies in human subjects
Level C-EO (expert opinion)
• The consensus of expert opinion based on clinical experience

Class of recommendation (COR) and level of evidence (LOE) are determined independently (any COR may be paired with any LOE). A recommendation with LOE C does not imply that the recommendation is weak. Many important clinical questions addressed in guidelines do not lend themselves to clinical trials. Although RCTs are unavailable, there may be a very clear clinical consensus that a specific test or therapy is useful or effective.
‡The method of assessing quality is evolving, including the application of standardized, widely used, and preferably validated evidence grading tools; and for systematic reviews, the incorporation of an Evidence Review Committee.
COR, class of recommendation; EO, expert opinion; LD, limited data; LOE, level of evidence; NR, nonrandomized; R, randomized; and RCT, randomized controlled trial.

Table 2.
Level (quality) of evidence‡ [131].

Telemedicine	COR	LOE
1. For sites without in-house imaging interpretation expertise, teleradiology systems approved by the US Food and Drug Administration are recommended for timely review of brain imaging in patients with suspected acute stroke.	I	A
2. When implemented within a telestroke network, teleradiology systems approved by the US Food and Drug Administration are useful in supporting rapid imaging interpretation in time for IV alteplase administration decision making.	I	A
3. Telestroke/teleradiology evaluations of acute ischemic stroke (AIS) patients can be effective for correct IV alteplase eligibility decision making.	IIa	B-R
4. Administration of IV alteplase guided by telestroke consultation for patients with AIS may be as safe and as beneficial as that of stroke centers.	IIb	B-NR
5. Providing alteplase decision-making support via telephone consultation to community physicians is feasible and safe and may be considered when a hospital has access to neither an in-person stroke team nor a telestroke system.	IIb	C-LD
6. Telestroke networks may be reasonable for triaging patients with AIS who may be eligible for interfacility transfer to be considered for acute mechanical thrombectomy.	IIb	B-NR

Table 3.
American Heart Association/American Stroke Association guidelines for telemedicine [131].

networks rely on real-time data sharing between the spoke and the hub, data security becomes a concern. Data security requires end-to-end encryption on the sharing platform, reliable documentation and storage, strict control of access to users within the network, and cooperation between the information technology staff at both sites. To ensure 24-hour coverage, consulting physicians often use a mobile device for such calls and must be cognizant of their surroundings while consulting remotely. For example, most telestroke systems provide home accessibility for physician consults. Currently due to HIPPA rules the use of hand held mobile phones remains limited for detection of stroke. Given the renewed interest in telehealth with the COVID-19 pandemic, there is a potential for use of mobile phone application technology.

Healthcare data breaches have been on the rise with larger and teaching hospitals being at a greater risk [132, 133]. Given multiple points of entry and the potential for data breaches in telestroke networks, extra care is needed at the hub and spokes sites to ensure data safety. Despite these challenges, telestroke networks have shown to provide safe, efficient, and cost-effective stroke care to underserved communities. There is still enormous potential for telestroke networks to expand into rural areas of the country as well as around the world.

11. Conclusion

Since its conception, telestroke has expanded greatly in its scope and utility in bridging the gap in stroke care between the rural and urban communities, in both acute and continued care. Despite the challenges faced in establishing and sustaining telestroke networks, these networks are flourishing and expanding, creating an ever-evolving paradigm for stroke care throughout the country and around the world.

Conflict of interest

The authors have no conflicts of interest to disclose.

Author details

Rohan Sharma[1], Krishna Nalleballe[1], Nidhi Kapoor[1], Vasuki Dandu[2], Karthika Veerapaneni[1], Sisira Yadala[1], Madhu Jasti[3], Suman Siddamreddy[2], Sanjeeva Onteddu[1] and Aliza Brown[1*]

1 Department of Neurology, University of Arkansas for Medical Sciences, Little Rock, AR, United States

2 Department of Neurology, Baptist Health Program, North Little Rock, AR, United States

3 Department of Neurology, University of Maryland Baltimore Washington Medical Center, Glen Burnie, MD, United States

*Address all correspondence to: brownalizat@uams.edu

References

[1] Grysiewicz RA, Thomas K, Pandey DK. Epidemiology of ischemic and hemorrhagic stroke: Incidence, prevalence, mortality, and risk factors. Neurologic Clinics. 2008;**26**(4): 871-895, vii

[2] Benjamin EJ et al. Heart disease and stroke statistics—2018 update: A report from the American Heart Association. Circulation. 2018

[3] Roger VL et al. Heart disease and stroke statistics—2011 update: A report from the American Heart Association. Circulation. 2011;**123**(4):e18-e209

[4] Rosamond W et al. Heart disease and stroke statistics—2007 update: A report from the American Heart Association Statistics Committee and Stroke Statistics Subcommittee. Circulation. 2007;**115**(5):e69-e171

[5] Saver JL et al. Time to treatment with intravenous tissue plasminogen activator and outcome from acute ischemic stroke. JAMA. 2013;**309**(23):2480-2488

[6] Mitka M. Early treatment of ischemic stroke with intravenous tPA reduces disability risk. JAMA. 2013;**310**(11):1111

[7] Meretoja A et al. Stroke thrombolysis: Save a minute, save a day. Stroke. 2014;**45**(4):1053-1058

[8] Nogueira RG et al. Thrombectomy 6 to 24 hours after stroke with a mismatch between deficit and infarct. The New England Journal of Medicine. 2018;**378**(1):11-21

[9] Albers GW et al. Thrombectomy for stroke at 6 to 16 hours with selection by perfusion imaging. The New England Journal of Medicine. 2018;**378**(8):708-718

[10] Berkhemer OA et al. A randomized trial of intraarterial treatment for acute ischemic stroke. The New England Journal of Medicine. 2015;**372**:11-20

[11] Jovin TG et al. Thrombectomy within 8 hours after symptom onset in ischemic stroke. The New England Journal of Medicine. 2015;**372**(24):2296-2306

[12] Fang MC, Cutler DM, Rosen AB. Trends in thrombolytic use for ischemic stroke in the United States. Journal of Hospital Medicine. 2010;**5**(7):406-409

[13] Katzan IL et al. Utilization of intravenous tissue plasminogen activator for acute ischemic stroke. Archives of Neurology. 2004;**61**(3):346-350

[14] Adeoye O et al. Recombinant tissue-type plasminogen activator use for ischemic stroke in the United States: A doubling of treatment rates over the course of 5 years. Stroke. 2011;**42**(7):1952-1955

[15] Prabhakaran S et al. Intravenous thrombolysis for stroke increases over time at primary stroke centers. Stroke. 2012;**43**(3):875-877

[16] Kleindorfer D et al. US geographic distribution of rt-PA utilization by hospital for acute ischemic stroke. Stroke. 2009;**40**(11):3580-3584

[17] Nalleballe K et al. Why are acute ischemic stroke patients not receiving thrombolysis in a telestroke network? Journal of Telemedicine and Telecare. 2019:1357633X18824518

[18] Leira EC et al. Rural-urban differences in acute stroke management practices: A modifiable disparity. Archives of Neurology. 2008;**65**(7):887-891

[19] Joubert J et al. Stroke in rural areas and small communities. Stroke. 2008;**39**(6):1920-1928

[20] Burgin WS et al. Acute stroke care in non-urban emergency departments. Neurology. 2001;**57**(11):2006-2012

[21] McConnell KJ et al. The on-call crisis: A statewide assessment of the costs of providing on-call specialist coverage. Annals of Emergency Medicine. 2007;**49**(6):727-733, 733.e1-733.e18

[22] Donnan GA, Davis SM. Neurologist, internist, or strokologist? Stroke. 2003;**34**(11):2765

[23] McConnell KJ, Newgard CD, Lee R. Changes in the cost and management of emergency department on-call coverage: Evidence from a longitudinal statewide survey. Annals of Emergency Medicine. 2008;**52**(6):635-642

[24] Rudkin SE et al. The state of ED on-call coverage in California. The American Journal of Emergency Medicine. 2004;**22**(7):575-581

[25] Goldstein LB et al. VA Stroke Study: Neurologist care is associated with increased testing but improved outcomes. Neurology. 2003;**61**(6):792-796

[26] Smith MA et al. 30-day survival and rehospitalization for stroke patients according to physician specialty. Cerebrovascular Diseases. 2006;**22**(1):21-26

[27] Zundel KM. Telemedicine: History, applications, and impact on librarianship. Bulletin of the Medical Library Association. 1996;**84**(1):71

[28] Bashshur R, Shannon GW. History of Telemedicine: Evolution, Context, and Transformation. New Rochelle, NY: Mary Ann Liebert; 2009

[29] Bashshur R, Lovett J. Assessment of telemedicine: Results of the initial experience. Aviation, Space, and Environmental Medicine. 1977;**48**(1):65-70

[30] Wittson CL, Benschoter R. Two-way television: Helping the medical center reach out. American Journal of Psychiatry. 1972;**129**(5):624-627

[31] Jutras A. Teleroentgen diagnosis by means of video-tape recording. The American Journal of Roentgenology, Radium Therapy, and Nuclear Medicine. 1959;**82**:1099-1102

[32] Grundy BL et al. Telemedicine in critical care: An experiment in health care delivery. JACEP. 1977;**6**(10):439-444

[33] Braly D. Telecom use grows for regional data access. Health Management Technology. 1995;**16**(7):22-24

[34] Levine SR, Gorman M. "Telestroke": The application of telemedicine for stroke. Stroke. 1999;**30**(2):464-469

[35] Hess DC, Audebert HJ. The history and future of telestroke. Nature Reviews Neurology. 2013;**9**(6):340

[36] Zachrison KS et al. Characterizing New England emergency departments by telemedicine use. The Western Journal of Emergency Medicine. 2017;**18**(6):1055

[37] Silva GS et al. The status of telestroke in the United States: A survey of currently active stroke telemedicine programs. Stroke. 2012;**43**(8):2078-2085

[38] Solenski NJ. Telestroke. Neuroimaging Clinics. 2018;**28**(4):551-563

[39] Demaerschalk BM et al. American Telemedicine Association: Telestroke guidelines. Telemedicine Journal and E-Health. 2017;**23**(5):376-389

[40] Holodinsky JK et al. Drip and ship versus direct to comprehensive stroke center: Conditional probability modeling. Stroke. 2017;**48**(1):233-238

[41] LaMonte MP et al. TeleBAT: Mobile telemedicine for the Brain Attack Team. Journal of Stroke and Cerebrovascular Diseases. 2000;**9**(3):128-135

[42] LaMonte MP et al. Shortening time to stroke treatment using ambulance telemedicine: TeleBAT. Journal of Stroke and Cerebrovascular Diseases. 2004;**13**(4):148-154

[43] Lippman JM et al. Mobile telestroke during ambulance transport is feasible in a rural EMS setting: The iTREAT Study. Telemedicine and e-Health. 2016;**22**(6):507-513

[44] Liman TG et al. Telestroke ambulances in prehospital stroke management: Concept and pilot feasibility study. Stroke. 2012;**43**(8):2086-2090

[45] Wu T-C et al. Telemedicine can replace the neurologist on a mobile stroke unit. Stroke. 2017;**48**(2):493-496

[46] Bowry R et al. Time to decision and treatment with tPA (tissue-type plasminogen activator) using telemedicine versus an onboard neurologist on a mobile stroke unit. Stroke. 2018;**49**(6):1528-1530

[47] Hacke W et al. Thrombolysis with alteplase 3 to 4.5 hours after acute ischemic stroke. The New England Journal of Medicine. 2008;**359**(13):1317-1329

[48] Wang S et al. Remote evaluation of acute ischemic stroke: Reliability of National Institutes of Health Stroke Scale via telestroke. Stroke. 2003;**34**(10):e188-e191

[49] Handschu R et al. Telemedicine in emergency evaluation of acute stroke: Interrater agreement in remote video examination with a novel multimedia system. Stroke. 2003;**34**(12):2842-2846

[50] Meyer BC et al. Reliability of site-independent telemedicine when assessed by telemedicine-naive stroke practitioners. Journal of Stroke and Cerebrovascular Diseases. 2008;**17**(4):181-186

[51] Demaerschalk BM, Kiernan T-EJ. Vascular neurology nurse practitioner provision of telemedicine consultations. International Journal of Telemedicine and Applications. 2010;**2010**

[52] Meyer B et al. Prospective reliability of the STRokE DOC wireless/site independent telemedicine system. Neurology. 2005;**64**(6):1058-1060

[53] Gonzalez MA et al. Reliability of prehospital real-time cellular video phone in assessing the simplified National Institutes of Health Stroke Scale in patients with acute stroke: A novel telemedicine technology. Stroke. 2011;**42**(6):1522-1527

[54] Demaerschalk BM et al. Reliability of real-time video smartphone for assessing National Institutes of Health Stroke Scale scores in acute stroke patients. Stroke. 2012;**43**(12):3271-3277

[55] Schwamm LH et al. A review of the evidence for the use of telemedicine within stroke systems of care: A scientific statement from the American Heart Association/ American Stroke Association. Stroke. 2009;**40**(7):2616-2634

[56] Puetz V et al. Reliability of brain CT evaluation by stroke neurologists in telemedicine. Neurology. 2013;**80**(4):332-338

[57] Demaerschalk BM et al. CT interpretation in a telestroke network: Agreement among a spoke radiologist, hub vascular neurologist, and hub neuroradiologist. Stroke. 2012;**43**(11):3095-3097

[58] Schwamm LH et al. Virtual TeleStroke support for the emergency department evaluation of acute stroke. Academic Emergency Medicine. 2004;**11**(11):1193-1197

[59] Wiborg A, Widder B. Teleneurology to improve stroke care in rural areas: The Telemedicine in Stroke in Swabia (TESS) Project. Stroke. 2003;**34**(12):2951-2956

[60] Hess DC et al. REACH: Clinical feasibility of a rural telestroke network. Stroke. 2005;**36**(9):2018-2020

[61] Wang S et al. Remote evaluation of acute ischemic stroke in rural community hospitals in Georgia. Stroke. 2004;**35**(7):1763-1768

[62] Joiner R et al. Abstract TP270: When telestroke programs work, bed size really doesn't matter. Stroke. 2019;**50**(Suppl_1):ATP270

[63] Switzer JA et al. A web-based telestroke system facilitates rapid treatment of acute ischemic stroke patients in rural emergency departments. The Journal of Emergency Medicine. 2009;**36**(1):12-18

[64] Audebert HJ et al. Effects of the implementation of a telemedical stroke network: The Telemedic Pilot Project for Integrative Stroke Care (TEMPiS) in Bavaria, Germany. The Lancet Neurology. 2006;**5**(9):742-748

[65] Demaerschalk BM et al. Cost utility of hub-and-spoke telestroke networks from societal perspective. The American Journal of Managed Care. 2013;**19**(12):976-985

[66] Nelson RE et al. The cost-effectiveness of telestroke in the treatment of acute ischemic stroke. Neurology. 2011;**77**(17):1590-1598

[67] Switzer JA et al. Cost-effectiveness of hub-and-spoke telestroke networks for the management of acute ischemic stroke from the hospitals' perspectives. Circulation. Cardiovascular Quality and Outcomes. 2013;**6**(1):18-26

[68] Nelson RE et al. The cost-effectiveness of telestroke in the Pacific Northwest region of the USA. Journal of Telemedicine and Telecare. 2016;**22**(7):413-421

[69] Ehlers L et al. National use of thrombolysis with alteplase for acute ischaemic stroke via telemedicine in Denmark. CNS Drugs. 2008;**22**(1):73-81

[70] Evans A et al. Randomized controlled study of stroke unit care versus stroke team Care in Different Stroke Subtypes. Stroke. 2002;**33**(2):449-455

[71] Wang DZ et al. Treating acute stroke patients with intravenous tPA: The OSF stroke network experience. Stroke. 2000;**31**(1):77-81

[72] Wiborg A, Widder B. Teleneurology to improve stroke care in rural areas. Stroke. 2003;**34**(12):2951-2956

[73] Vespa PM et al. Intensive care unit robotic telepresence facilitates rapid physician response to unstable patients and decreased cost in neurointensive care. Surgical Neurology. 2007;**67**(4):331-337

[74] Klein KE et al. Teleneurocritical care and telestroke. Critical Care Clinics. 2015;**31**(2):197-224

[75] Laver KE et al. Telerehabilitation services for stroke. Cochrane Database of Systematic Reviews. 2013;**12**:1-41

[76] Chen J et al. Telerehabilitation approaches for stroke patients: Systematic review and meta-analysis of randomized controlled trials. Journal of Stroke and Cerebrovascular Diseases. 2015;**24**(12):2660-2668

[77] Blacquiere D et al. Canadian stroke best practice recommendations: Telestroke best practice guidelines update 2017. International Journal of Stroke. 2017;**12**(8):886-895

[78] Switzer JA et al. A telestroke network enhances recruitment into acute stroke clinical trials. Stroke. 2010;**41**(3):566-569

[79] Kramer NM, Demaerschalk BM. A novel application of teleneurology: Robotic telepresence in supervision of neurology trainees. Telemedicine and e-Health. 2014;**20**(12):1087-1092

[80] Jagolino AL et al. A call for formal telemedicine training during stroke fellowship. Neurology. 2016;**86**(19):1827-1833

[81] Richard S et al. Simulation training for emergency teams to manage acute ischemic stroke by telemedicine. Medicine. 2016;**95**(24):e3924

[82] Rafter RH, Kelly TM. Nursing implementation of a telestroke programme in a community hospital in the US. Journal of Nursing Management. 2011;**19**(2):193-200

[83] Zaidi SF et al. Telestroke-guided intravenous tissue-type plasminogen activator treatment achieves a similar clinical outcome as thrombolysis at a comprehensive stroke center. Stroke. 2011;**42**(11):3291-3293

[84] Huynh MNN et al. Abstract 173: Effect of a regional telestroke program on door-to-needle time and clinical outcomes. Stroke. 2019;**50**(Suppl_1):A173

[85] Donabedian A. The quality of care: How can it be assessed? JAMA. 1988;**260**(12):1743-1748

[86] Schwamm LH et al. Get With the Guidelines—Stroke is associated with sustained improvement in care for patients hospitalized with acute stroke or transient ischemic attack. Circulation. 2009;**119**(1):107-115

[87] Yang JP et al. Targeting telestroke: Benchmarking time performance in telestroke consultations. Journal of Stroke and Cerebrovascular Diseases. 2013;**22**(4):470-475

[88] Meyer BC et al. Efficacy of site-independent telemedicine in the STRokE DOC trial: A randomised, blinded, prospective study. The Lancet Neurology. 2008;**7**(9):787-795

[89] Amorim E et al. Impact of telemedicine implementation in thrombolytic use for acute ischemic stroke: The University of Pittsburgh Medical Center telestroke network experience. Journal of Stroke and Cerebrovascular Diseases. 2013;**22**(4):527-531

[90] Nalleballe K et al. Ideal telestroke time targets: Telestroke-based treatment times in the United States stroke belt. Journal of Telemedicine and Telecare. 2020;**26**(3):174-179

[91] Schwab S et al. Long-term outcome after thrombolysis in telemedical stroke care. Neurology. 2007;**69**(9):898-903

[92] Wechsler LR et al. Telemedicine quality and outcomes in stroke: A scientific statement for healthcare professionals from the American Heart Association/American Stroke Association. Stroke. 2017;**48**(1):e3-e25

[93] LaMonte MP et al. Telemedicine for acute stroke: Triumphs and pitfalls. Stroke. 2003;**34**(3):725-728

[94] Whitten P, Love B. Patient and provider satisfaction with the use of telemedicine: Overview and rationale for cautious enthusiasm. Journal of Postgraduate Medicine. 2005;**51**(4):294

[95] National Quality Forum (NQF) Stroke Prevention and Management. National Voluntary Consensus Standards for Stroke Prevention and Management across the Continuum of Care. A Consensus Report. Washington, DC: NQF; 2009:1-13

[96] Brown A et al. A pilot study validating video-based training on pre-hospital stroke recognition. Journal of Neurology, Neurosurgery, and Psychiatry Research. 2019;**1**(1):1-12

[97] Fassbender K et al. Streamlining of prehospital stroke management: The golden hour. The Lancet Neurology. 2013;**12**(6):585-596

[98] Baldereschi M et al. Relevance of prehospital stroke code activation for acute treatment measures in stroke care: A review. Cerebrovascular Diseases. 2012;**34**(3):182-190

[99] Belvís R et al. Benefits of a prehospital stroke code system. Cerebrovascular Diseases. 2005;**19**(2):96-101

[100] Burton A. How do we fix the shortage of neurologists? The Lancet Neurology. 2018;**17**(6):502-503

[101] Agarwal S et al. Thrombolysis delivery by a regional telestroke network—Experience from the UK National Health Service. Journal of the American Heart Association. 2014;**3**(1):e000408

[102] Sairanen T et al. Two years of Finnish telestroke: Thrombolysis at spokes equal to that at the hub. Neurology. 2011;**76**(13):1145-1152

[103] Ohannessian R et al. Acute telestroke in France: A systematic review. Revue Neurologique. 2020;**176**(5):316-324

[104] Muller-Barna P et al. TeleStroke units serving as a model of care in rural areas: 10-year experience of the TeleMedical project for integrative stroke care. Stroke. 2014;**45**(9):2739-2744

[105] Audebert HJ et al. Long-term effects of specialized stroke care with telemedicine support in community hospitals on behalf of the Telemedical Project for Integrative Stroke Care (TEMPiS). Stroke. 2009;**40**(3):902-908

[106] Hubert GJ et al. Recommendations on telestroke in Europe. European Stroke Journal. 2019;**4**(2):101-109

[107] Zhao G, Huang H, Yang F. The progress of telestroke in China. Stroke and Vascular Neurology. 2017;**2**(3):168-171

[108] Sharma S et al. Telestroke in resource-poor developing country model. Neurology India. 2016;**64**(5):934

[109] Srivastava PV et al. Telestroke a viable option to improve stroke care in India. International Journal of Stroke. 2014;**9**(SA100):133-134

[110] Imai T et al. Specific needs for telestroke networks for thrombolytic therapy in Japan. Journal of Stroke and Cerebrovascular Diseases. 2014;**23**(5):811-816

[111] Ang SH, Tan C, Singh R. Telestroke: Rapid treatment of acute ischemic stroke patients using telemedicine in a Singapore emergency department. European Journal of Emergency Medicine. 2013;**20**(5):322-326

[112] Rho MJ, Choi IY, Lee J. Predictive factors of telemedicine service acceptance and behavioral intention of physicians. International Journal of Medical Informatics. 2014;**83**(8):559-571

[113] Wu Z, McGoogan JM. Characteristics of and important lessons from the coronavirus disease

2019 (COVID-19) outbreak in China: Summary of a report of 72 314 cases from the Chinese Center for Disease Control and Prevention. JAMA. 2020;**323**(13):1329-1242

[114] Cucinotta D, Vanelli M. WHO declares COVID-19 a pandemic. Acta Biomed. 2020;**91**(1):157-160

[115] Characteristics of Health Care Personnel with COVID-19—United States, February 12–April 9, 2020. Available from: https://www.cdc.gov/mmwr/volumes/69/wr/mm6915e6.htm?s_cid=mm6915e6_x [Accessed: 16 April 2020]

[116] Klok F et al. Incidence of thrombotic complications in critically ill ICU patients with COVID-19. Thrombosis Research. 2020;**191**:145-147

[117] Hollander JE, Carr BG. Virtually perfect? Telemedicine for Covid-19. The New England Journal of Medicine. 2020;**382**(18):1679-1681

[118] Klein BC, Busis NA. COVID-19 is catalyzing the adoption of teleneurology. Neurology. 2020;**94**(21):903-904

[119] Reider-Demer M et al. Tele neurology-cost effective and convenient (1205). AAN Enterprises. Science Highlight Virtual Presentations. Cerebrovascular Disease and Interventional Neurology; 2020

[120] Trevino A et al. Inpatient teleneurology follow-up has similar outcomes to in-person neurology and provides an alternative to transfer (1861). AAN Enterprises. Science Highlight Virtual Presentations. Cerebrovascular Disease and Interventional Neurology; 2020

[121] Aita MC et al. Obstacles and solutions in the implementation of telestroke: Billing, licensing, and legislation. Stroke. 2013;**44**(12):3602-3606

[122] Weinstein RS et al. Telemedicine, telehealth, and mobile health applications that work: Opportunities and barriers. The American Journal of Medicine. 2014;**127**(3):183-187

[123] Akbik F et al. Telestroke—The promise and the challenge. Part two—Expansion and horizons. Journal of Neurointerventional Surgery. 2017;**9**(4):361-365

[124] Audebert HJ, Schwamm L. Telestroke: Scientific results. Cerebrovascular Diseases. 2009;**27**(Suppl 4):15-20

[125] Cho S et al. An analysis of business issues in a telestroke project. Journal of Telemedicine and Telecare. 2007;**13**(5):257-262

[126] De Bustos EM, Moulin T, Audebert HJ. Barriers, legal issues, limitations and ongoing questions in telemedicine applied to stroke. Cerebrovascular Diseases. 2009;**27**(Suppl. 4):36-39

[127] Rogove HJ et al. Barriers to telemedicine: Survey of current users in acute care units. Telemedicine and e-Health. 2012;**18**(1):48-53

[128] Switzer JA, Demaerschalk BM. Overcoming challenges to sustain a telestroke network. Journal of Stroke and Cerebrovascular Diseases. 2012;**21**(7):535-540

[129] Joint Commission on Accreditation of Healthcare Organizations. Joint Commission realigns telemedicine requirements with CMS changes. Joint Commission Perspectives. 2011;**31**(10):6

[130] Schwamm LH et al. Recommendations for the implementation of telemedicine within stroke systems of care: A policy statement from the American Heart Association. Stroke. 2009;**40**(7):2635-2660

[131] Powers WJ et al. 2018 guidelines for the early management of patients with acute ischemic stroke: A guideline for healthcare professionals from the American Heart Association/ American Stroke Association. Stroke. 2018;**49**(3):e46-e99

[132] Kamoun F, Nicho M. Human and organizational factors of healthcare data breaches: The swiss cheese model of data breach causation and prevention. International Journal of Healthcare Information Systems and Informatics (IJHISI). 2014;**9**(1):42-60

[133] Bai G, Jiang JX, Flasher R. Hospital risk of data breaches. JAMA Internal Medicine. 2017;**177**(6):878-880

Section 2

Treatment of Ischemic Stroke

Chapter 5

The Treatment of Acute Stroke

Irina Alexandrovna Savvina and Anna Olegovna Petrova

Abstract

Stroke is a major public health issue, because of its high incidence rate, high case fatality rate, risk of residual physical and neuropsychological disabilities, and direct and indirect costs. Many strokes are preventable and treatable in the acute stage, provided that patients are admitted soon enough. The term stroke covers a wide range of heterogeneous disorders, depending on the severity of the clinical presentation, from transient deficits to severe cases with coma and early death; the underlying mechanism, i.e., cerebral ischemia, parenchymal hemorrhage, subdural hemorrhage, or subarachnoid hemorrhage (SAH); and the cause, i.e., atherosclerosis, cardioembolism, small-vessel occlusion, rare vasculopathies and undetermined causes in cerebral ischemia, or vascular malformations, cerebral amyloid angiopathies, small-vessel diseases, rare vasculopathies and undetermined causes in parenchymal hemorrhages. This chapter will focus only on acute cerebral ischemia and parenchymal hemorrhage. We will cover the general assessment of stroke patients, the complications that can occur in the acute stage, the treatment of acute stroke, and finally a few situations that require specific managements and where evidence-based data are scarce.

Keywords: cerebral ischemia, parenchymal hemorrhages, thrombolytic therapy, complications

1. Introduction

This chapter focuses on the treatment of acute cerebral ischemia and intracranial hemorrhage, which are two types of stroke. Stroke is characterized by a sudden loss of brain function with no established cause other than vascular origin. This applies to both ischemic stroke and intracranial hemorrhage.

1.1 The diagnosis of stroke

Acute stroke suggests the following signs:

- Sudden onset of symptoms and development of the clinical picture in a few seconds or minutes with further stabilization or improvement.

- Focal neurological symptoms associated with damage to certain parts of the brain: motor deficits (weakness or immobility of the limbs on one side of the body (hemiplegia or hemiparesis) or an isolated limb), loss of sensitivity (decreased sensitivity in various parts of the body), aphasia, agnosia, and vision disorders.

- Symptoms suggesting a loss of function: limb tremors, convulsions, paresthesias, visual hallucinations, and flashes before the eyes.

- Headache, nausea and vomiting, dysphagia, dysarthria, dysphonia, diplopia, ataxia, hiccups, one-sided acute hearing loss, respiratory disorder, convulsive syndrome, and transient loss of consciousness may be clinical manifestations of a stroke localized in the brain stem.

- Symptoms such as loss of consciousness, dizziness, general weakness, confusion, urinary incontinence, syncopal condition, and tinnitus do not indicate the development of a stroke if they are not associated with focal neurological symptoms.

For the differential diagnosis of ischemic and hemorrhagic strokes, it is necessary to conduct a neuroimaging study [1]. This is the most important stage of diagnosis, because patients with ischemic and hemorrhagic strokes require different therapies in the acute period and various measures of secondary prevention [2].

Magnetic resonance imaging (MRI) is the most appropriate diagnostic method for patients with acute cerebral circulation disorders due to the following reasons [3]:

1. T1- and T2-weighted images and fluid-attenuated inversion recovery (FLAIR) sequences allow the differentiation of old foci and foci of nonvascular origin.

2. Diffusion-weighted images allow the identification of new ischemic foci. Low brain blood flow causes the development of cytotoxic cell edema and, as a result, a decrease in the movement of extracellular fluid, which is displayed as a hyperintensive signal on diffusion-weighted images, and a decrease in the water diffusion coefficient. These changes appear earlier than changes in T1 and T2 and FLAIR.

3. T* sequences are used to detect hemorrhages.

4. Time-of-flight (TOF) MR angiography can be used to visualize the occlusion of extra- and intracranial arteries.

When MRI is not available in an emergency or cannot be performed due to contraindications (established rhythm driver, claustrophobia, psychomotor agitation), an emergency computed tomography (CT) scan of the brain is performed without contrast. CT scan reveals an intracranial hemorrhage in the form of a hyperintensive zone in the brain parenchyma. **Figure 1** shows a non-contrast CT scan with a spontaneous hyperdensity of the right cerebral hemisphere, due to a deep intracerebral hemorrhage (ICH). In the early stages of acute cerebral ischemia, CT signs of ischemia may be absent. But within 3 hours, you can see signs of ischemia, for example, the disappearance of a clear border of gray and white matter. With the occlusion of the middle cerebral artery, CT signs will appear in the form of a hyperintensive zone. CT with contrast allows you to visualize the anatomy of the arteries and perfusion.

The most common causes of ischemic stroke are common atherosclerosis, atrial fibrillation (AF), occlusion of small perforating arteries of the brain, pathology of heart valves, and infectious diseases, in young patients—cerebral artery dissection.

Intracerebral hemorrhages in most cases are the result of the damage to small cerebral vessels due to chronic arterial hypertension or amyloid angiopathy.

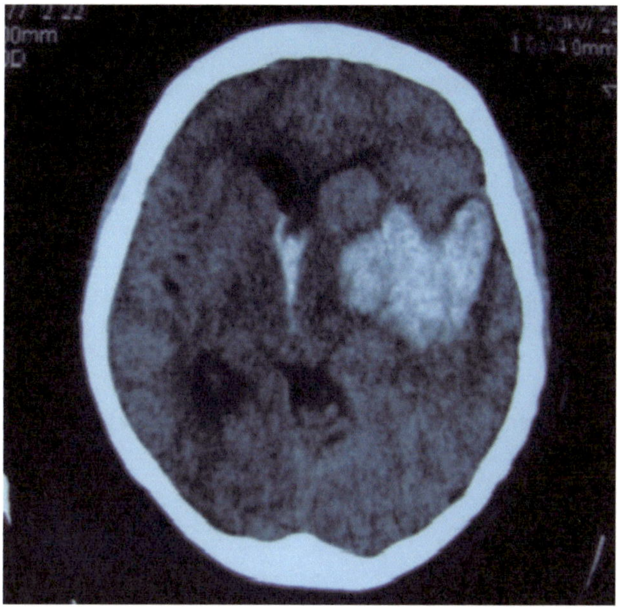

Figure 1.
Non-contrast CT scan shows a spontaneous hyperdensity of the right cerebral hemisphere.

1.2 Examination of patients with acute stroke

For all patients in the acute stage, the following examinations should be carried out, which will determine the treatment plan: a thorough collection of anamnesis to determine the presence of hypertension, medications used, alcohol abuse, and substance abuse and a family history of stroke, oncology, and trauma; a clinical examination; blood test to detect polycythemia and plateletemia, erythrocyte sedimentation rate (ESR) to detect vasculitis, and the level of glycemia to detect diabetes or hypoglycemia, and coagulation tests. Cardiac assessment including electrocardiogram (ECG) and echocardiography (EchoCG) is quite important in all cases and Holter in selected cases. ECG recording to detect heart attacks, atrial fibrillation, continuous ECG monitoring to detect arrhythmias; monitoring of systolic, diastolic, and mean blood pressure (BP) by noninvasive method; dopplerography to detect stenoses and dissections of cervical and intracranial vessels; transthoracic EchoCG to detect blood clots, tumors, valve pathology, vegetations on the valves, reduction of ejection fraction, and the presence of an open oval window. Neuroimaging methods include MRI and CT of the brain to detect caverns, intracranial venous thromboses, cerebral microhemorrhages, arteriovenous malformations (AVM), tumors, and indirect signs of unknown injuries. Additional examinations are prescribed depending on the initial results obtained, the patient's age, and the presumed etiology of the stroke: angiography (usually MR, CT angiography) and specific biological tests when it comes to specific causes, such as antinuclear antibodies, etc.

There are neurological complications that occur in the acute phase of stroke in any type in the form of convulsive syndrome; hyper- and hypoactive delirium, especially with a pre-existing decrease of cognitive functions and the development of metabolic or infectious complications; as well as intracranial hypertension.

Nonspecific complications include bedsores, pneumonia, urinary tract infection, hyponatremia due to inadequate secretion of antidiuretic hormone (ADH), deep vein thrombosis, and pulmonary thromboembolism. They are more likely to develop in patients with severe neurological deficits. Hyponatremia is a common accompaniment during the acute stage of stroke. Its relevance to the clinical presentation, treatment and prognosis should be mentioned.

1.2.1 Protocol of hypernatremia correction in patients with stroke

Hypernatremia: Na >145 mmol/l (the main reason—central DI)
Criteria: polyuria: rate of diuresis >3 ml/kg/hour
Hypernatremia: >145 mmol/l
Urine specific gravity: <1005

Infusion therapy:

Base 75–100 ml/hour monitoring of sodium concentration every 6 hours.
Fluid deficit replenishment: in case of polyuria—compensation of fluid loss.

If ineffective, symptoms of diabetes insipidus (DI) persist—ADH

Desmopressin: 2–4 mcg per 24 hours
Vasomirin (nasal spray): 10 mcg

1.2.1.1 Fluid loss calculation

Total body fluid = 0.6 × body weight
Free water deficit = (0.6 × body weight) − (0.6 × body weight) × (140/Na act)
Example: body weight = 75 kg, Na = 154 mmol/l
Free water deficit = 0.6 × 75 − [0.6 × 75 × (140/154)] = 45 − 40.9 = 4.1 l

1.2.2 Protocol of hyponatremia correction in patients with stroke

Hyponatremia: Na < 135 mmol/l
If Na <125 mmol/l, there is a high risk of neurological disorders.

1. Syndrome of inappropriate antidiuretic hormone secretion (SIADH)

    A. No neurological deterioration

    B. Acute neurological deterioration

    - Hyponatremia: no longer than 24 hours acute not prolonged reducing the level of sodium
    - Negative fluid balance: IV 3% NaCl—4 ml/kg during 15–30 min
    - 2/3 of physiological need for fluid + furosemide 1 mg/kg
    - Intravenous (IV): only sodium solutions
    - Monitoring: fluid balance, diuresis, sodium in plasma/urine, and urine specific gravity

2. Central salt wasting syndrome

A. Restoring of fluid deficit

B. Positive sodium balance

C. Rehydration

D. HyperHAES: 0.25 ml/kg/hour or 0.9%NaCl

E. Fludrocortisone: 0.4 mg per 24 hours

F. Acute hyponatremia correction rate (<48 h): ≤24 mmol/l/24 hours

G. Chronic hyponatremia correction rate (>48 h): ≤0.5 mmol/l/hour, but ≤10 mmol/l/24 hours

H. In the presence of an accompanying potassium deficit: ≤4 mmol/l/25 hours

2. Treatment of acute stroke

2.1 General principles of the therapy

Stroke patients should be treated in specialized departments. For every 24 patients treated in a specialized rather than general ward, one death and one disability are prevented [4]. This does not depend on the age, type, and severity of stroke [4, 5]. Therefore, specialized departments are very important for the treatment of stroke patients [1, 4]. For all strokes with persistent neurological deficits, the treatment aimed at stabilizing the patient's condition, controlling vital functions, and actively curating problems that may worsen recovery is indicated. This is the main component of the stroke treatment program [6, 7].

In the detection and treatment of emergency life-threatening conditions (risk of aspiration, epileptic status, respiratory failure, etc.), the patency of the upper respiratory tract should be ensured in the case of deprivation of consciousness to the level of coma, respiratory failure of central origin, or local causes leading to respiratory disorders.

The stabilization of most physiological parameters, blood pressure, saturation (more than 93%), glycemic level (less than 180 mg), body temperature (below 37.50°C), and hydration, is necessary in the first few days to prevent negative dynamics in the penumbra zone.

A normal respiratory function with adequate blood oxygenation is necessary in the acute period of stroke to maintain an adequate oxygen delivery to brain cells, but there is no conclusive evidence that all patients with stroke receive oxygen therapy with a positive result [4]. In cases of hypoxemia, improved blood oxygenation is achieved by oxygen therapy via a nasal catheter and noninvasive or invasive ventilation.

Complications of acute stroke include neurogenic stressful cardiomyopathy, paroxysmal sympathetic hyperactivity, atrial fibrillation, acute heart failure, myocardial infarction, and sudden death [1, 2]. The frequency of these complications explains the need for a constant monitoring for 2–3 days.

Many stroke patients are in a state of dehydration, which leads to a worse outcome of the disease [1, 2]. Despite limited clinical data, the administration of infusion therapy (0.9% sodium chloride solution) is considered part of the overall treatment of stroke, especially in patients with an increased risk of dehydration due to depression of consciousness or respiratory disorders. Experience in the treatment of hyperglycemia recommends avoiding the introduction of glucose solutions in the early period of stroke and strict control of the level of glycemia [4].

According to the literature, there are no mechanisms for autoregulation of cerebral blood flow in the penumbra zone. Therefore, a decrease in blood pressure in the first hours after a stroke before the penumbra zone appears can cause significant hypoperfusion, which worsens the development of the ischemia zone. Therefore, in the acute period, it is not necessary to aggressively treat arterial hypertension if there are no concomitant life-threatening conditions, such as aortic dissection or intracranial hematoma [2, 4].

In practice, blood pressure correction is usually started when the systolic blood pressure exceeds 220 mm Hg and diastolic blood pressure exceeds 120 mm Hg. However, in many clinics, antihypertensive therapy is performed only in cases of heart failure, acute renal failure, aortic arch dissection, or malignant hypertension. When conducting a thrombolytic therapy (TLT), it is common practice to maintain blood pressure below 185 mm Hg. The intravenous administration of labetalol (10 mg bolus, followed by an infusion of 0.1–0.3 mg/kg/hour) or urapidil (12.5 mg bolus for 20 seconds, followed by an infusion of 6–30 mg/hour) is often used.

Hyperglycemia occurs in 60% of stroke patients who have not previously suffered from diabetes [2, 7]. Hyperglycemia after a stroke is usually associated with a large volume of infarction and cortical damage and is associated with an adverse outcome of the disease [4]. Currently, the routine use of insulin infusions in patients with moderate hyperglycemia is not recommended. The European Stroke Association recommends maintaining glycemia below 180 mg/dl (10 mmol/l) [4].

Body temperature control: hyperthermia is associated with an increase in the size of the infarction zone and a worsening of the outcome of the disease [8]. Fever is associated with a worse clinical outcome [9]. When the body temperature increases, it is necessary to quickly exclude concomitant infections and, if necessary, treat them.

2.1.1 Prevention of acute stroke complications

The prevention of trophic disorders in the form of bedsores is carried out by establishing an early enteral nutrition through a nasogastric probe with an adequate calorie of nutritional mixtures: early mobilization, anti-bedsore mattresses, suitable beds, and nursing care.

Aspiration pneumonia: diagnosis of dysphagia (special examination of the function of swallowing by doctors, nurses, or speech therapists) [10, 11] or use of a nasogastric probe if necessary.

Deep vein thrombosis and pulmonary embolism: low-molecular-weight heparins (LMWH) in prophylactic doses reduce the risk of thromboembolic complications without affecting mortality [2]. Their use slightly increases the risk of intracranial hemorrhages. The use of LMWH is recommended only if the patient has risk factors for deep vein thrombosis and pulmonary embolism, such as lower limb immobilization, in the first few hours after a stroke [2], and not earlier than 24 hours in patients with intracranial hemorrhage [9]. A recent study of Clots in Legs Or sTockings after Stroke (CLOTS) [12] has shown that an intermittent pneumatic compression reduces the risk of deep vein thrombosis and can improve stroke survival in patients who cannot go to the toilet with an assistant.

Rehabilitation: it is an important issue both in acute phase and in chronic phase. Points to be covered are position turning to avoid pressure sores, chest physiotherapy to minimize lung complication, swallowing assessment and training, limb movements to prevent deep vein thrombosis, speech therapy, early mobilization, etc. All should be started as early as possible. Rehabilitation should begin as soon as the patient's condition stabilizes: passive measures to minimize contractures, bedsores, and pneumonia. A coordinated multidisciplinary approach to patient management with the help of constantly trained staff is important, which leads to a reduction in mortality and disability.

2.2 Thrombolytic therapy

The intravenous administration of a recombinant tissue plasminogen activator (tPA) increases the chances of a favorable outcome approximately 8 times within 3 months if performed in the first 90 minutes, 2 times when performed within 91–180 minutes after a stroke, and 1.4 times when performed in 181–270 minutes [6, 13]. The mortality does not change when administered up to 270 min after stroke onset, but increases with later administration of tPA [6]. Indications and contraindications for thrombolytic therapy are noted in **Tables 1** and **2**, respectively.

Hemorrhagic transformation is more often observed in patients with large strokes and of old age [7]. The earlier the tPA is introduced, the more likely the beneficial effect is, and despite the fact that the probability of a favorable effect is also present when used later than 3 hours from a stroke, it is significantly reduced. The dose is 0.9 mg/kg (10% intravenous bolus, 90%—within an hour microjet). In Japan, the recommended dose is lower—0.6 mg/kg. Thus, thrombolytic therapy is recommended as early as possible after the onset of a stroke, no later than 4.5 hours. Restrictions apply both to contraindications [increased risk of hemorrhage, delay of more than 4.5 hours, blood pressure (BP) above 185 mm Hg, blood glucose above 4 G/l] and strict rules of use (only by a doctor trained in the management of stroke patients and only in the stroke department) [6].

Other ways to achieve rapid recanalization are currently being investigated and do not change the existing recommendations: other thrombolytic drugs, MRI patient selection criteria, intra-arterial thrombolytic therapy, and ultrasound-assisted intravenous thrombolysis. Mechanical thrombextraction is considered a promising technique in addition to intravenous thrombolysis in patients with proximal occlusions. In patients receiving oral anticoagulants, mechanical thrombectomy is often the only recommended recanalization strategy.

2.3 Antithrombotic therapy

Aspirin at a starting dose of 300 mg and then 75–150 mg daily prevents 9 cases of disability and death per 1000 patients. Aspirin should be prescribed 24 hours after any thrombolytic therapy. Recently, a Clopidogrel in High-Risk Patients with Acute Nondisabling of Cerebrovascular Events (CHANCE) study showed that patients with small strokes and transient ischemic attack (TIA) who received a loading dose of clopidogrel for 24 hours, against the background of aspirin, and then for 90 days on 75 mg of aspirin and 75 mg of clopidogrel had better outcomes without the risk of bleeding.

No. of wording
1. Stroke, ischemic type
2. The time from the symptoms onset to the thrombolysis procedure less than 4.5 hours
3. Age from 18 years and older (after 80 years with caution, individual decision about TLT, taking into account the perceived risk)

Table 1.
Indications for thrombolytic therapy.

No. of wording
Cerebral
1. Neuroimaging (CT, MRI) signs of intracranial hemorrhages, brain tumors
2. Hemorrhagic stroke or stroke of an unspecified nature in the anamnes
3. Rapid improvement or mild symptoms by the time of the beginning of TLT (non-invalidizing symptoms) in the absence of data for occlusion of the main vessels
4. Signs of a severe stroke: clinical [score on the National Institutes of Health Stroke Scale (NIHSS) > 25), neuroimaging (based on CT of the brain and/or MRI of the brain in the diffusion-weighted imaging (DWI) mode, the focus of ischemia extends to the territory of a larger basin medium cerebral artery (MCA)]
5. Convulsions at the beginning of a stroke (if there is reason to assume that focal symptoms are represented by Todd's paresis)
6. Previous stroke or severe traumatic brain injury within 3 months
7. Suspected subarachnoid hemorrhage (SAH)
8. Surgical intervention on the brain or spinal cord in the anamnesis
Cerebral and somatic
9. Arterial aneurysms, defects in the development of arteries or veins
10. Tumors with a high risk of bleeding
Somatic
11. Hypersensitivity to any component of the drug
12. Hemorrhagic diathesis
13. Arterial hypertension over 185/110 mm Hg or necessity in intensive reduction of less than these figures
14. Bacterial endocarditis, pericarditis
15. Gastrointestinal or urogenital bleeding during the last 3 weeks. Confirmed exacerbations of peptic ulcer disease of the stomach and duodenum during the last 3 months
16. Liver failure (cirrhosis, active hepatitis, portal hypertension)
17. Acute pancreatitis
18. Present bleeding or extensive bleeding in the recent 6 months
19. Extensive surgery, trauma, delivery, puncture of large vessels, cardiopulmonary resuscitation within the last 10 days
20. Recent myocardial infarction
21. Pregnancy
22. Data on bleeding or acute injury (fracture) at the time of examination
Laboratory
23. Taking indirect anticoagulants (warfarin) if international normalized ratio (INR) >1.3
24. Use of heparin for 48 hours with increased activated partial thromboplastin time (aPTT)
25. Thrombocytopenia less than 100,000/mm^3
26. Glycemia less than 2.8 and more than 22.5 mmol/l
27. With previous administration of new oral anticoagulants (dabigatran, rivaroxaban, apixaban), indicators of aPTT, INR, quantity of platelets, thrombin time, or Xa factor activity should be within normal values. In the absence of the ability to determine the laboratory data, the last intake of a drug from the oral anticoagulant group should be >2 days before the development of stroke (with normal kidney function)
28. Other diseases or conditions with increased risk of bleeding or other complications of TLT (the decision is made by the council of physicians)

Table 2.
Contraindications for thrombolytic therapy.

Low-molecular-weight heparins do not have advantages, because a decrease in the frequency of early recurrent strokes is balanced by an increase in the frequency of hemorrhagic transformations. There is no reason to recommend heparin in the acute stage of ischemic stroke, even in patients with atrial fibrillation.

2.4 Hypothermia and neuroprotection

Experimental studies have shown that potential neuroprotectors are effective, but this is not confirmed in the human population. Many neuroprotective agents have been developed based on a cascade of biochemical events leading to cell death.

We report below the current clinical status of drugs that have been developed as neuroprotective agents (**Table 3**) [14].

Hypothermia is a potential opportunity to provide neuroprotection, but due to side effects and the need for intensive therapy, it can only be used in severe cases, especially in patients with malignant heart attacks, and currently requires randomized trials [8, 15].

2.5 Decompressive neurosurgery

Decompressive neurosurgery (hemispherectomy) reduces mortality and disability in patients younger than 60 years old who recently suffered a massive stroke

Category, mechanism	Drug name, name of multicenter study, and its results	Category, mechanism	Drug name, name of multicenter study, and its results
Ca^{2+} channel blocker	Nimodipine: no benefit (VENUS)	Noncompetitive NMDA antagonist	Dizocilpine, discontinued Dextrorphan, no benefit
Na^{+} channel blocker	Lifarizine, no benefit; lubeluzole, no benefit; fosphenytoin, discontinued	Competitive NMDA antagonist	Selfotel: discontinued
GABA agonist	Clomethiazole: no effect	AMPA/KA receptor antagonist	NBQX, discontinued YM872, RCT
Free radical scavenger	Edaravone, clinical use; ebselen, phase III; NXY059: phase III; tirilazad, discontinued	Metabotropic receptor antagonist	Groups I, II, and III: RCT being planned
Growth factor	bFGF: abandoned AX200 (filgrastim, G-CSF analogue), phase II	LMWH-CoA reductase inhibitor	Lovastatin, phase II; simvastatin, phase III
Growth factors, oxygen delivery	Human chorionic gonadotropin (hCG)/erythropoietin (Ntx-265): phase II	Hemodiluting agent	Albumin: phase III (ALIAS)
Ganglioside	No benefit	Membrane stabilizer	Citicoline (CDP choline): phase III
$MgSO_4$	FAST-MAG: ongoing (IMAGE)	Iron chelator	Deferoxamine mesylate: phase II
Opioid receptor antagonist	Nalmefene: no benefit	Metal ion chelator	DP-b99: phase III
Polyamine receptor antagonist	Eliprodil: discontinued	Antibiotic, pleiotropic protective effects	Minocycline: phase III
Glycine antagonist	ACEA-1021, no benefit; gavestinel, no benefit	Others	Piracetam: phase III

VENUS, very early nimodipine use in stroke; NMDA, N-methyl-D-aspartic acid; GABA gamma-aminobutyric acid; AMPA, amino-hydroxy-methyl-isoxalone propionic acid; KA, kainate; NBQX, 2,3dihydroxy-6-nitro-7-sulfamoyl-benzo [f]quinoxaline-2,3-dione; RCT, randomized controlled trial; bFGF basic fibroblast growth factor; ALIAS, albumin in acute stroke; FAST-MAG, Field Administration of Stroke Therapy—Magnesium; ACEA-1021, 5-nitro-6,7-dichloro-1,4dihydro-2,3-quinoxalinedione.

Table 3.
Neuroprotective drugs developed so far and results of clinical trials.

in the middle cerebral artery basin [16]. In order to be effective, the operation must be performed before the development of a malignant brain attack. The best selection criterion is the volume of damage on a diffusion-weighted MRI within 24 hours; a volume greater than 145 cm^3 is a good predictor of malignant infarction. Therefore, the best candidates for surgical treatment are patients younger than 60 years with a lesion volume of more than 145 cm^3 on diffusion-weighted MRI (6.50). The effectiveness of hemispherectomy is great—every second death is prevented. Results of the Decompressive Surgery for the Treatment of Malignant Infarction of the Middle Cerebral Artery II (DESTINY II) study also showed effectiveness in patients over 60 years of age [3].

3. Treatment of intracranial hemorrhage

It is necessary to control blood pressure (BP). Lowering blood pressure in the first hours can prevent or slow down the growth of hematoma, as well as reduce the risk of repeated hemorrhage.

An early decrease in blood pressure can cause cerebral ischemia in low-perfused and hypometabolic regions of the brain adjacent to the hematoma.

European recommendations are based on the evidence of a low level of significance (class 4) [9]:

- No specific drug is recommended.

- In patients with a history of primary arterial hypertension or signs (ECG, changes in the fundus vessels) of chronic hypertension, systolic pressure above 180 mm Hg or diastolic pressure above 105 mm Hg and in patients without a history of hypertension, the target blood pressure is 170/100 or average 125 mm Hg.

- In patients without a history of arterial hypertension (systolic blood pressure above 160 mm Hg and/or diastolic blood pressure above 95 mm Hg), the target blood pressure is 150/90 mm Hg or BP mean 110 mm Hg.

- Avoid lowering blood pressure by more than 20%. These targets should be revised for patients who are being monitored for intracranial pressure (ICP) and are experiencing intracranial hypertension in order to maintain adequate cerebral perfusion pressure (greater than 70 mm Hg).

The INTERACT 2 study recently showed that in patients with intracerebral hematoma, an intensive reduction in blood pressure with targets below 140 mm Hg within an hour slightly improves the outcome and is well tolerated by the patient.

3.1 Prevention of deep vein thrombosis and pulmonary embolism

In patients with intracerebral hematoma, complications such as deep vein thrombosis and pulmonary embolism are feared. A small study conducted on patients with intracerebral hematoma showed that the use of intermittent pneumatic compression is more effective than the use of compression knitwear alone [17]. The CLOTS study [12] showed that the use of compression knitwear is ineffective, but only 232 patients with intracerebral hematoma were included out of 2518 stroke patients. The expediency of using heparin and low-molecular-weight heparins is justified only in cases where the probability of bleeding risk is less than the possible benefit of prescribing drugs. In clinical practice, low doses of fractionated or low-molecular-weight heparin can be prescribed after 24 hours [16]. According to the results of the CLOTS 3 study [12], intermittent pneumatic compression is effective.

3.2 Intracranial hypertension

ICP negatively affects the functional outcome. The superiority of invasive ICP monitoring over clinical observation and neuroimaging has not been proven. Ways to reduce ICP by medication help to buy time to prepare for surgical decompression, if it is planned. In the acute phase of intracranial hemorrhage, it is recommended to avoid corticosteroids. These recommendations are based on low confidence data. For the medical treatment of ICH, glycerol, mannitol, HAES, and short-term hyperventilation (confidence class 4) are used. For example, mannitol (20%) at a dose of 0.75–1.0 g/kg can be administered as an intravenous bolus followed by 0.25–0.5 g/kg every 3–6 hours, depending on the neurological status and fluid balance.

3.3 Intracranial hemorrhage in patients receiving oral anticoagulants

In the acute stage, every patient with intracranial hemorrhage and an INR greater than 1.4 should receive intravenous vitamin K and drugs that replace the deficiency of clotting factors, despite the reason for taking oral anticoagulants (including patients with artificial valves). The goal is to prevent the growth of hematoma volume. In European protocols, it is recommended to use a concentrated prothrombin complex or SPP together with the intravenous administration of vitamin K [18]. Doses of concentrated prothrombin complex: 10–20 U/kg, if the INR is less than 3.5; or 20–30 units/kg, if the INR exceeds 3.5; together with 10 mg of vitamin K in/B.

Recombinant factor VIIa is not recommended for routine use outside of clinical trials.

There is currently no antidote for patients with intracranial hematoma receiving new oral anticoagulants. This limits the use of these drugs.

There are no specific recommendations for the treatment of hemorrhage on the background of antiplatelet drugs. Studies of the use of thrombosis have not proved its effectiveness [6, 13].

3.4 Thrombolytic therapy

In patients with intracranial hemorrhage with increased ventricles and obstruction of the third and fourth ventricles, according to some data, it is recommended to use a recombinant tissue plasminogen activator inserted directly into the ventricular system, which can improve the functional outcome [9].

3.5 Neurosurgical intervention

The removal of a blood clot should be considered in cases where there is neurological dysfunction or neuroimaging data about occlusion of cerebrospinal fluid spaces subtentorially. According to European recommendations, ventricular drainage and hematoma removal should be performed when the size of the hematoma is more than 2–3 cm in diameter or in the presence of hydrocephalus, even if the favorable outcome is doubtful due to old age or coma.

Dynamic monitoring and conservative medical treatment are the first stage in the treatment of patients with intracranial hematoma. A special analysis of subgroups from the STICH study and a recent meta-analysis showed that craniotomy should be considered as a treatment option in cases of depression of consciousness (from 12 to 9 points on the Glasgow scale) [19] or in cases of superficial intracranial hemorrhage (less than 1 cm from the surface and does not reach the basal ganglia) [20–22]. With deep-seated hematomas, craniotomy does not bring a positive result. The STICH II study showed that early surgical treatment did not increase mortality and disability within 6 months, but slightly improved survival in patients with spontaneous intracranial hemorrhage in the absence of intraventricular hemorrhage.

4. Specific clinical situations

4.1 Treatment of stroke due to sinus thrombosis

Sinus thrombosis is the cause of approximately 1% of strokes. It occurs due to the occlusion of the venous sinuses and/or cortical veins. This can lead to a venous infarction with petechial hemorrhages or a perivascular venous infarction. Usually, the cause of sinus thrombosis is congenital and acquired prothrombotic disorders, such as pregnancy and infections, including infections of the central nervous system as well as ear, sinuses, mouth, face, or neck. Also the predisposing factors are various diagnostic and therapeutic procedures, such as surgery, lumbar puncture, jugular vein catheterization, and administration of certain medications, especially oral contraceptives, hormone replacement therapy, steroids, and antitumor drugs [23].

The clinical picture may be different, but sinus thrombosis should be excluded in young patients with recent headache and stroke-like symptoms, transient neurological deficits, convulsions, or lobar intracranial hemorrhages. This is especially true for patients with intracranial hypertension and patients with signs of hemorrhagic infarctions, especially if they are numerous and correspond to certain vascular pools.

The gold standard for diagnosing sinus thrombosis is MRI, which provides direct visualization of occluded veins, sinuses, and blood clots [23]. Sometimes CT is used for diagnostics, but if MRI is available, this is not the method of choice for diagnostics. On CT, you can see a hyperintensive shadow of a blood clot in the occluded sinus, the so-called cord symptom.

4.1.1 Heparin therapy

The available research data on the treatment of venous thrombosis recommend the use of heparin, as it reduces the risk of death and severe disability without the risk of intracranial hematoma. It has been shown that anticoagulant therapy leads to an absolute reduction in the risk of death and disability by 13% and a relative reduction in the risk by 54%, as well as a positive effect of using heparin without increasing the risk of intracranial hemorrhage.

According to European recommendations [18], venous thrombosis should be treated with low-molecular-weight heparins subcutaneously or intravenous heparin; doses are selected by body weight. The presence of intracranial hemorrhage accompanying venous thrombosis is not a contraindication to a heparin therapy [18].

4.1.2 Thrombolytic therapy

There is no data from randomized controlled trials on the efficacy and safety of systemic or local thrombolytic therapy in patients with cerebral vein thrombosis and sinus thrombosis. A recently published systematic review of thrombolytic therapy in patients with cerebral vein thrombosis and sinus thrombosis suggests a favorable effect in comatose patients [24].

According to European protocols [18], there is insufficient data to recommend the use of systemic or local thrombolytic therapy in patients with cerebral vein thrombosis and sinus thrombosis. Thrombolytic therapy may be an option if the patient's condition worsens despite an adequate anticoagulant therapy.

4.1.3 Oral anticoagulants

After the acute phase, they switch to oral anticoagulant therapy. The Target INR is 2.0–3.0. In cases of cerebral vein thrombosis and sinus thrombosis during pregnancy, oral anticoagulants are not prescribed due to their possible teratogenic effects and the ability to penetrate the placenta. In these cases, anticoagulant therapy is continued with heparin. There is no available data from controlled studies concerning the optimal duration of anticoagulant therapy in patients with cerebral vein thrombosis and sinus thrombosis. MRI data from 33 patients showed that recanalization occurs within 4 months after cerebral vein thrombosis and sinus thrombosis, regardless of further anticoagulation therapy [25].

According to European protocols [18], anticoagulants can be prescribed for 3 months if cerebral vein thrombosis occurred due to transient factors and for 6–12 months in patients with idiopathic thrombosis and congenital "moderate" thrombophilia.

4.1.4 Anticonvulsant therapy

The preventive use of anticonvulsants is controversial. Some studies have shown that sensory and motor deficits, parenchymal lesions on MRI/CT, and cortical vein thrombosis can be independent predictors of early symptomatic epileptic seizures [26]. According to European recommendations [18], prophylactic administration of anticonvulsants is possible for patients with local neurological deficits and foci of parenchymal lesions. Treatment can be continued for a year. Despite the fact that 50% of patients with venous thrombosis experience brain edema, mild edema can be relieved by isolated administration of heparin to restore venous outflow. Steroids are not recommended for the treatment of intracranial hypertension due to their unproven effectiveness. In severe cases, with the threat of transtentorial dislocation, surgical decompression is considered the only lifesaving method of treatment.

4.2 Cardiac surgery and strokes

The incidence of strokes in the postoperative period in patients with coronary artery bypass grafting (CABG) is about 2%, and a higher incidence of strokes is observed in patients after valve replacement operations and other cardiac surgeries [3]. The causes of stroke after cardiac surgery include perioperative embolism from the aortic arch or heart chambers, systemic hypoperfusion, ischemia associated with occlusion of large vessels, or a combination of these factors [3]. Risk factors for stroke after cardiac surgery are old age; a history of strokes, hypertension, and diabetes mellitus; the presence of noise in the projection of the carotid arteries; the use of bronchodilators and diuretics; high serum creatinine levels; recovery of large vessels; the use of inotropes after artificial circulation; and the duration of artificial blood circulation.

Currently, there are no special recommendations for the treatment of patients with stroke after CABG [3]. Moreover, patients with stroke after CABG are treated as patients with acute stroke with loading doses of aspirin (160–320 mg) [3].

4.3 Operations on the carotid arteries and strokes

Carotid endarterectomy is the standard method for treating carotid artery stenosis [3]. It is recommended for 70–99% of patients with symptomatic stenosis. It is confirmed that surgical treatment of asymptomatic stenosis reduces the risk of ipsilateral stroke; however, the absolute advantage of this method has not been proven. Currently, stenting is not recommended for revascularization of the carotid arteries.

The pathophysiological mechanism of stroke in carotid revascularization may be associated with hemodynamic cerebral ischemia or arterio-arterial embolism. The latter mechanism may be more frequent during stenting due to endovascular access.

4.4 Acute coronary syndrome (ACS) and stroke

Intracranial hemorrhage can be a severe side effect of thrombolytic therapy in ACS. The risk of intracranial hemorrhage depends on the previous episodes in the history, age, and mode of thrombolytic therapy. Usually, the risk of intracranial hemorrhage during thrombolytic therapy of acute myocardial infarction is 0.5–1%.

There are no special recommendations for the treatment of ischemic stroke in ACS in European protocols. In the presence of ACS, the protocols of the European Stroke Organization recommend lowering blood pressure [4, 6]. An anticoagulant therapy is not recommended, while a combination of clopidogrel and aspirin is recommended in terms of cardiac causes [4, 7].

4.5 Stroke in patients with atrial fibrillation

Cardio-cerebral embolism is considered to be the cause of at least 20% of ischemic strokes, and non-valvular AF is the most common cause, associated with a fivefold increase in the risk of stroke, and accounts for 25% of all strokes in patients older than 80 years [3]. Long-term thromboprophylaxis is necessary to prevent strokes in patients with AF. Recently, for patients who cannot be treated with warfarin and clopidogrel, it has been shown that clopidogrel and aspirin therapy reduces the risk of vascular accidents [7]. Oral direct thrombin inhibitors such as dabigatran have been shown to be effective in preventing stroke and systemic embolism with a risk of intracranial hemorrhage comparable to that of warfarin. Stroke in patients with AF can be divided into three groups:

1. Ischemic stroke in patients with insufficient therapy, i.e., not receiving anticoagulants, despite scores on the CHADS2 scale greater than 2 [3]

2. Ischemic stroke that developed despite warfarin therapy

3. Intracranial hemorrhage that occurred in a patient receiving anticoagulants

The incidence of intracranial hemorrhage increases 7–10 times compared to patients who do not receive oral anticoagulants and is 1.8% per year in patients at risk of stroke [7].

4.5.1 Treatment

In the acute phase of stroke, heparin is not recommended; its use leads to a slight decrease in repeated strokes, an indefinite decrease in mortality, and a disability with an increase in the frequency of intracranial hemorrhages [7].

4.6 Cerebrocardial syndrome (neurogenic stress cardiomyopathy)

The connection between the brain and the heart reflects a complex multidirectional complex regulation of systemic hemodynamics and organ autoregulation of local perfusion, which is especially pronounced in a cerebral catastrophe. Arrhythmias, in particular AF, often accompany the development of stroke, while myocardial infarction, Takotsubo syndrome, and sudden death are rare, although they are also described in strokes [27–29]. Sometimes stroke patients are found to have high levels of troponin, indicating myocardial damage.

5. Conclusion

To ensure adequate treatment, a rapid diagnosis of stroke and its nature and cause is necessary. Specialized stroke departments allow for effective treatment and specific therapy.

Conflict of interest

The authors declare no conflict of interest.

Notes/thanks/other declarations

We would like to thank our teachers—neurologists, anesthesiologists, and neurosurgeons—of Russian Polenov's Neurosurgical Institute, the first institute of neurological surgery in the world founded in 1926 in St. Petersburg (Petrograd) in Russia.

Abbreviations

ACS	acute coronary syndrome
AF	atrial fibrillation
ADH	antidiuretic hormone
aPTT	activated partial thromboplastin time
AVM	arteriovenous malformation
BP	blood pressure
CT	computed tomography
CABG	coronary artery bypass grafting
DI	diabetes insipidus
DWI	diffusion-weighted imaging
ECG	electrocardiogram
EchoCG	echocardiography
ESR	erythrocyte sedimentation rate
LMWH	low-molecular-weight heparins

ICH	intracranial hemorrhage
ICP	intracranial pressure
INR	international normalized ratio
MCA	medium cerebral artery
MRI	magnetic resonance imaging
NIHSS	National Institutes of Health Stroke Scale
SAH	subarachnoid hemorrhage
SIADH	syndrome of inappropriate antidiuretic hormone secretion
tPA	tissue plasminogen activator
TLT	thrombolytic therapy

Author details

Irina Alexandrovna Savvina[1,2] and Anna Olegovna Petrova[1]*

1 Almazov National Medical Research Centre of Ministry of Health of Russian Federation, Saint Petersburg, Russia

2 Mechnikov State North-West Medical University, Saint Petersburg, Russia

*Address all correspondence to: petrovaanna2803@gmail.com

References

[1] Cordonnier C, Leys D. Stroke: The bare essentials. Practical Neurology. 2008;**8**:263-272. DOI: 10.1136/jnnp.2008.149401

[2] Hankey GJ, Warlow CP. Treatment and secondary prevention of stroke: Evidence, costs, and effects on individuals and populations. Lancet. 1999;**354**:1457-1463

[3] Leys D, Cordonnier C, Caso V. Stroke. In: Tubaro M, Vranckx P, Price S, Vrints C, editors. The ESC Textbook of Intensive and Acute Cardiovascular Care. 2nd ed. Oxford, UK: Oxford University Press; 2015. pp. 645-656. DOI: 10.1093/med/9780199687039.001.0001

[4] Georgiadis D, Schwab S. Hypothermia in acute stroke. Current Treatment Options in Neurology. 2005; 7:119-127

[5] Adams HP Jr, Bendixen BH, Kappelle LJ, et al. Classification of subtype of acute ischemic stroke. Definitions for use in a multicenter clinical trial. TOAST. Trial of Org 10172 in Acute Stroke Treatment. Stroke. 1993;**24**:35-41. DOI: 10.1161/01.STR.24.1.35

[6] Hacke W, Kaste M, Bluhmki E, et al. Thrombolysis with alteplase 3 to 4.5 hours after acute ischemic stroke. The New England Journal of Medicine. 2008;**359**:1317-1329

[7] Warlow C, van Gijn J, Dennis M, et al. Stroke: Practical Management. 3rd ed. Oxford: Blackwell Science; 2008

[8] European Stroke Organisation Working Group. Guidelines for management of ischaemic stroke and transient ischaemic attack 2008. Cerebrovascular Diseases. 2008;**25**:457-507. DOI: 10.1159/000131083

[9] Steiner T, Kaste M, Forsting M, et al. Recommendations for the management of intracranial haemorrhage—Part I: Spontaneous intracerebral haemorrhage. The European Stroke Initiative Writing Committee and the Writing Committee for the EUSI Executive Committee. Cerebrovascular Diseases. 2006;**22**:294-316

[10] Bussell SA, González-Fernández M. Racial disparities in the development of dysphagia after stroke: Further evidence from the medicare database. Archives of Physical Medicine and Rehabilitation. 2011;**92**(5):737-742

[11] Splaingard ML, Hutchins B, Sulton LD, et al. Aspiration in rehabilitation patients: Videofluoroscopy vs bedside clinical assessment. Archives of Physical Medicine and Rehabilitation. 1988; **69**(8):637-640

[12] Dennis M, Sandercock P, Graham C, Forbes J. The Clots in Legs or sTockings after Stroke (CLOTS) 3 trial: A randomised controlled trial to determine whether or not intermittent pneumatic compression reduces the risk of post-stroke deep vein thrombosis and to estimate its cost-effectiveness. Health Technology Assessment. 2015;**19**(76). DOI: doi.org/10.3310/hta19760

[13] Hacke W, Brott T, Caplan L, et al. Thrombolysis in acute ischemic stroke: Controlled trials and clinical experience. Neurology. 1999;**53**:S3-S14

[14] Murozono M. Neuroprotective drugs. In: Uchino H, Ushijima K, Ikeda Y, editors. Neuroanesthesia and Cerebrospinal Protection. Japan: Springer; 2015. pp. 119-126. DOI: 10.1007/978-4-431-54490-6

[15] Bart van der Worp H, Macleod MR, Kollmar R. Therapeutic hypothermia for acute ischemic stroke: Ready to start

large randomized trials? Journal of Cerebral Blood Flow and Metabolism. 2010;**30**(6):1079-1093. DOI: 10.1038/jcbfm.2010.44 Jгащищен

[16] Vahedi K, Hofmeijer J, Juettler E, et al. Early decompressive surgery in malignant infarction of the middle cerebral artery: A pooled analysis of three randomised controlled trials. Lancet Neurology. 2007;**6**:215-222

[17] Sachdeva A, Dalton M, Amaragiri SV, Lees T. Graduated compression stockings for prevention of deep vein thrombosis. Cochrane Database of Systematic Reviews. Dec 2014;(12):CD001484. DOI: 10.1002/14651858.CD001484.pub3

[18] Duranteau J, Taccone FS, Verhamme P, et al. For the ESA VTE Guidelines Task Force. European guidelines on perioperative venous thromboembolism prophylaxis. Intensive care. European Journal of Anaesthesiology. 2018;**35**:142-146. DOI: 10.1097/EJA.0000000000000702

[19] Kim JE, Ko S-B, Kang H-S, et al. Clinical practice guidelines for the medical and surgical management of primary intracerebral hemorrhage in Korea. Journal of Korean Neurosurgical Association. 2014;**56**(3):175-187. DOI: 10.3340/jkns.2014.56.3.175

[20] Rost NS et al. Prediction of functional outcome in patients with primary intracerebral hemorrhage: The FUNC score. Stroke. 2008;**39**(8): 2304-2309

[21] Hemphill JC, Bonovich DC, Besmertis L, Manley GT, Johnston SC. The ICH Score: A simple, reliable grading scale for intracerebral hemorrhage. Stroke. 2001;**32**:891-897

[22] Clarke JL, Johnston SC, Farrant M, Bernstein R, Tong D, Hemphill JC. External validation of the ICH score. Neurocritical Care. 2004;**1**(1):53-60

[23] Tadi P, Babak Behgam B, Baruffi S. Cerebral Venous Thrombosis [Internet]. StatPearls Publishing. 2020. Available from: https://www.ncbi.nlm.nih.gov/books/NBK459315/ [Accessed: 16 March 2020]

[24] Viegas L, Viegas LD, Stolz E, Canhão P, Ferro JM. Systemic thrombolysis for cerebral venous and dural sinus thrombosis: A systematic review. Cerebrovascular Diseases. 2014; **37**:43-50. DOI: doi.org/10.1159/000356840

[25] Caso V, Agnelli G, Paciaroni M, editors. Handbook on Cerebral Venous Thrombosis. Frontiers of Neurology and Neuroscience. Vol. 23. Basel, Karger. 2008. pp. I-VI. DOI: 10.1159/isbn.978-3-8055-8379-4

[26] Habibabadi JM, Mohammad Saadatni M, Tabrizi N. Seizure in cerebral venous and sinus thrombosis. Epilepsia Open. 2018;**3**(3):316-322. DOI: 10.1002/epi4.12229

[27] Weiner MM, Asher DI, Augoustides JG, et al. Takotsubo cardiomyopathy: A clinical update for the cardiovascular anesthesiologist. Journal of Cardiothoracic and Vascular Anesthesia. 2017;**31**(1):334-344. DOI: 10.1053/j.jvca.2016.06.004

[28] Belkin AA, Gromov VS, Levit AL, et al. Cerebrocardial syndrome. Differential diagnostic, treatment tactics. Anesthesiologia and Reanimatologia. 2012;**4**:81-85. (In Russ.) ISSN: 2410-4698 (Online), 0201-7563 (Print), ISSN-L 0201-7563

[29] Kato K, Lyon AR, Ghadri J-R, et al. Takotsubo syndrome: Aetiology, presentation and treatment. Heart. 2017;**103**:1461-1469. DOI: 10.1136/heartjnl-2016-309783

Chapter 6

Vinpocetine and Ischemic Stroke

Hayder M. Al-kuraishy and Ali I. Al-Gareeb

Abstract

Vinpocetine (VPN) is a synthetic ethyl-ester derivative of the alkaloid apovincamine from *Vinca minor* leaves. VPN is a selective inhibitor of phosphodiesterase type 1 (PDE1) has potential neurological effects through inhibition of voltage gated sodium channel and reduction of neuronal calcium influx. VPN have noteworthy antioxidant, anti-inflammatory and anti-apoptotic effects with inhibitory effect on glial and astrocyte cells during and following ischemic stroke (IS). VPN is effective as an adjuvant therapy in the management of epilepsy; it reduces seizure frequency by 50% in a dose of 2 mg/kg/day. VPN improves psychomotor performances through modulation of brain monoamine pathway mainly on dopamine and serotonin, which play an integral role in attenuation of depressive symptoms. VPN recover cognitive functions and spatial memory through inhibition of hippocampal and cortical PDE-1with augmentation of cAMP/cGMP ratio, enhancement of cholinergic neurotransmission and inhibition of neuronal inflammatory mediators. Therefore, VPN is an effective agent in the management of ischemic stroke and plays an integral role in the prevention and attenuation of post-stroke epilepsy, depression and cognitive deficit through direct cAMP/cGMP-dependent pathway or indirectly through anti-inflammatory and anti-oxidant effects.

Keywords: vinpocetine, phosphodiesterase type 1, antioxidant, anti-inflammatory, stroke, post-stroke

1. Introduction

Vinpocetine (VPN) is a synthetic ethyl-ester derivative of the alkaloid apovincamine from *Vinca minor* leaves which is known as lesser periwinkle. A VPN has a specific chemical structure contains carboxylic acid ethyl ester which is soluble in alcohol, acetone and sulfoxide, **Figure 1** [1].

VPN is widely used in the treatment of different cerebro-vascular disorders, cognitive dysfunction, memory disorders, tinnitus, macular degeneration and glaucoma. In addition, VPN is effective in the management of acute kidney injury, renal stone, hair loss and peptic ulceration [2].

Nevertheless, this critical review only focused on the potential role of VPN in the management of ischemic stroke.

A multiplicity of search strategies was taken and assumed which included electronic database searches of Medline and Pubmed using MeSH terms, keywords and title words during the search. The terms used for these searches were as follows: [Vinpocetine OR apovincamine] AND [cognitive function OR stroke OR brain ischemia OR blood flow OR cerebral circulation OR oxidative stress OR blood

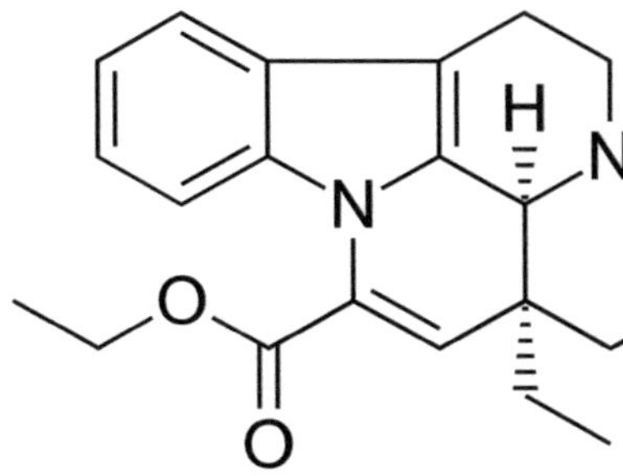

Figure 1.
Chemical structure of Vinpocetine.

viscosity OR cerebral blood flow]. [Vinpocetine OR apovincamine] AND [cerebral metabolism OR cerebral hypoxia OR ischemic degeneration OR minor stroke]. Reference lists of identified and notorious articles were reviewed. In addition, only English articles were considered and case reports were not concerned in the review. The key features of recognized applicable search studies were considered and the conclusions summarized in a critical review.

2. Pharmacology of vinpocetine

VPN is a selective inhibitor of phosphodiesterase type 1 (PDE1) which increasing of cAMP and cGMP leading to vasodilatation. Also, it inhibits the release of pro-inflammatory cytokines through inhibition of IKK/NF-kB activator protein-1 (AP-1) pathway which is involved in the propagation of inflammatory cytokines translocation and release [3]. Moreover, VPN has potential neurological effects through inhibition of voltage gated sodium channel, reduction of neuronal calcium influx and antioxidant effect with augmentation of dopamine metabolism since it increases 3, 4-dihydroxyphenylacetic acid (DOPAC) which is the breakdown metabolites of dopamine [4].

It has been reported that VPN is a safe drug for long-term use and it well tolerated during the management of cerebrovascular disorders. Mild side effects such as headache, flushing, anxiety, dry mouth and nausea have been accounted during VPN uses. In spite of potent non-selective vasodilator effect it does not produce stealing effect on cerebral vasculatures due to the viscosity lowering effect and inhibition of platelet aggregations which together improve cerebral vessels rheological properties. Nevertheless, VPN does not reduce blood pressure and systemic circulation during acute and chronic uses [5].

VPN is well absorbed from small intestine, which increased by food, therefore, fasting bioavailability is 6.7% and non-fasting bioavailability is 60–100%. Similarly, VPN has no significant drug-drug interactions with different drugs such as oxazepam, imipramine, glibenclamide and other agents that are used in the management of ischemic stroke [6].

3. Vinpocetine in ischemic stroke

Ischemic stroke (IS) represents the main leading cause of death in the American Unite State and developed countries and regarded it as the main cause of long-term disability. IS represents 11.9% of annual total death and accounts for 90% of all stroke cases [7]. Arboix study discussed briefly the risk factor of IS [8]. These risk factors are divided into non-modifiable risk factors (sex, age, inherited factors, ethicinity and low birth weight at birth) and modifiable risk factors (diabetes mellitus, hypertension, smoking, obesity, alcohol abuse, oral contraceptive and metabolic syndrome). [9] IS is mainly caused by arterial thrombosis on the atherosclerotic plaque of cerebral vessels, causing cerebral ischemia, infarction and induction of peri-infarct inflammation. Neuro-inflammations contribute into tissue repair and neuronal damage as well as retrograde and anterograde axonal degenerations [10]. IS leads to glucose and oxygen deprivation of neuronal cells which causing oxidative stress, excitotoxicity and calcium overload which eventually causing neuronal cell death and development of infarction core [11]. The infracted core and damaged neuronal cells due to induced oxidative stress, releasing of various inflammatory molecules that causing vasculitis and damage of blood brain barrier (BBB) [12]. Moreover, activated microglia and infiltrated macrophage during IS release neurotransmitters which are interact with neurons causing neuroinflammation and neuronal injury. As well, interleukin-8(IL-8), NF-kB and tumor necrosis factor (TNF-α) are over-expressed during IS which play a potential role in the initiation of inflammation and apoptosis [13]. In a similar way, vascular smooth muscle and endothelial cells of cerebral vasculature are activated by NF-kB pathway leading to further obstruction and thrombosis. Therefore, NF-kB pathway is an important pathway in the pathogeneses and development of neurological deficit thus; inhibition of NF-kB pathway by VPN is regarded as important and main mechanism of VPN neuroprotection [14].

In addition, activated microglia expresses cholesterol transporter protein (TSPO) which is over-expressed during brain injury and IS and inhibited by VPN [15].

During IS voltage gated sodium channels are activated causing intracellular accumulation of Na and Ca leading to neuronal cell damage, excitotoxicity, edema, acidosis and acute cellular dysfunctions. VPN inhibits voltage gated sodium channels leading to dose dependent reduction of intracellular concentrations of Na and Ca. Thus, the neuroprotective effect of VPN during IS is chiefly mediated by inhibition of neuronal voltage gated sensitive Na-channel [16].

Different studies illustrated that oxidative stress, excitotoxicity and impaired energy metabolism leading to neuronal death by both apoptosis and necrosis during IS. These events lead to reduction of cAMP system which is important in the expression and regulation of brain derived neurotrophic factor (BDNF), which improves neuronal survival. PDE1 is mainly localized in striatum and cortex which participating in the regulation of neuronal motor activity [17, 18].

Indeed, VPN increases neuronal cGMP through inhibition of calmodulin dependent phosphodiesterase which improves cerebral blood flow and oxygen consumption [19]. VPN improves cerebral metabolism through enhancing glucose and oxygen supply and ATP production by cerebral vasodilation. These effects prevent IS induced-memory and cognitive dysfunctions due to improvement of neurotransmitters such as serotonin, dopamine and noradrenaline, which are involved in the regulation of cognitive function [20].

3.1 Antioxidant effects of vinpocetine in ischemic stroke

In IS overproduction of free radicals and reactive oxygen and/or nitrogen species lead to neuro-pathological changes through complex interactions with cellular components such as proteins, DNA and lipids. Free radicals, mainly superoxide and non-radicals such as hydrogen peroxide may cause further neurological injury through depletion of endogenous antioxidant capacity. Therefore, drug with antioxidant potential may play a role in the prevention of cerebral injury during IS [21].

Recent study by Al-Kuraishy et al. reported that VPN is a potent antioxidant agent which improves antioxidant capacity and reduces of oxidative stress [22]. As well, Santos et al., study illustrated that VPN attenuates oxidative stress during IS through inhibition of lipid peroxidation and generation of free radical [23]. In addition, VPN has a potential neuroprotective effect, though antioxidant effect since it prevents oxidative stress injury and toxic demyelination in rat brain [24]. The antioxidant neuroprotective effect of VPN is mainly at low-moderate doses since; high doses of VPN lead to oxidative stress due to prooxidant and proinflammatory effects [25]. Deshmukh et al. reported that antioxidant potential of VPN contributes into the prevention of IS induced-neuronal injury through modulation of cholinergic neurons [26]. Therefore, antioxidant mechanisms of VPN are related to direct free radical scavenging effect, potentiating of endogenous antioxidant capacity and inhibition the generation of free radicals. The molecular antioxidant effect of VPN is linked to the suppression of ADP stimulated respiration, mitochondrial Na+/Ca+ exchange, mitochondrial swelling and regulation of mitochondrial membrane potentials [16, 27].

3.2 Anti-inflammatory effects of vinpocetine in ischemic stroke

IS induced-inflammatory changes and neuroinflammations lead to secondary brain damage. Toll-like receptors (TLRs) are over-expressed in IS, leading to the induction the release of pro-inflammatory mediators through myeloid differentiation factor-88 (MyD88) dependent pathway and Toll /IL-IR domain-containing adaptor factor protein inducing interferon-beta (TRIF) dependent pathway [28]. Therefore, inhibition of TLR4/MyD88 and NF-$_{K}$B pathways lead to noteworthy neuroprotection against IS. It has been noted that VPN inhibits TNF-α induced NF-$_{K}$B activation, pro-inflammatory releases and inflammatory biomarkers such as

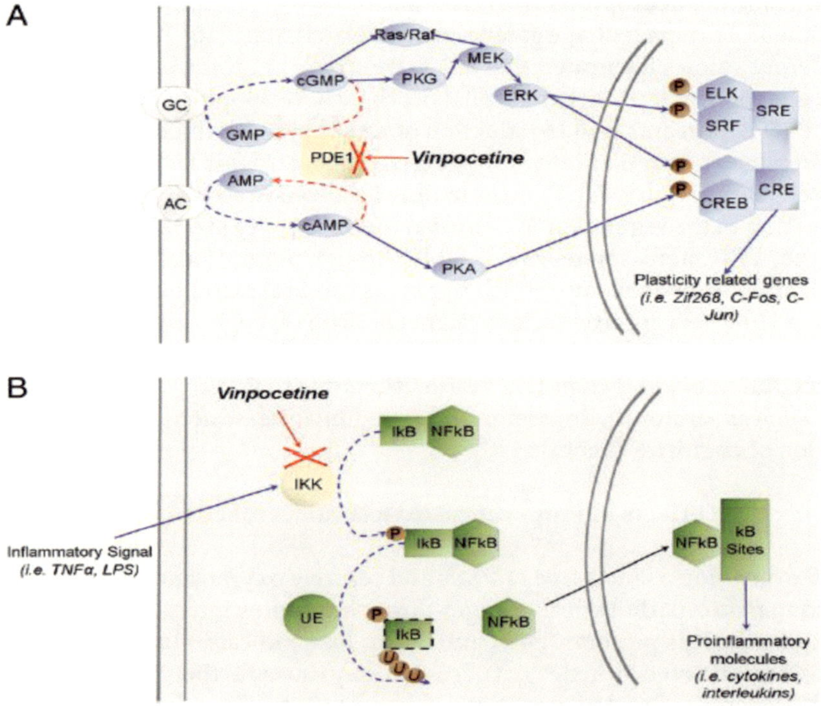

Figure 2.
Anti-inflammator effects of vinpocetine. (A) Basic effect, (B) Anti-inflammatory effect.

IL-1β and IL-33 in an experimental ischemic model [5]. In intriguing way, Zhang and Yang reported that VPN inhibits the release of chemokines and inflammatory cytokines from microglia, macrophage and endothelial cells in IS through inhibition of NF-$_{K}$B pathways in IS and associated atherosclerosis [29]. In a similar way, VNP leads to the significant neuroprotective effect and regulation of neuronal plasticity through the anti-inflammatory effect which is mediated by suppression of IB-Kinase (IKK) pathway in IS, **Figure 2** [30, 31].

Usually, microglia cells are resident macrophages in the brain and act as an active immune defense against cerebral injury and infection through induction and regulation of neuro-inflammatory reactions. Microglia improves brain homeostasis through removal of tissue debris, dead cells, and induction of neurogenesis and preservation of myelin sheath with secretion of neuroprotective factors such as insulin-like growth factor. On the other hand, activated microglia leads to neuronal injury during IS through the release of TNF-α, IL-6, IL1β and nitric oxide (NO) [32]. It has been reported that VPN inhibits neuronal inflammation in IS through suppression of microglia activity [33]. Also, VPN inhibits IS induced-inflammatory changes and reduces brain edema and infarction size mainly through inhibition the expression of NF-$_{K}$B and TNF-α in the activated microglia which is PDE1 independent pathway [34].

3.3 Effects of vinpocetine on ischemic reperfusion injury in ischemic stroke

Ischemic-reperfusion (I/R) injury in IS leads to activations of perivascular macrophages, which play a role in the progression of neuronal damage through the release of proinflammatory biomarkers which also participate in the injury to blood brain barrier. Furthermore, activate macrophages, microglia, T-cells and dendritic cells infiltrate the infarct site following I/R injury causing further damage through the release of monocyte chemoattracting protein (MCP-1) which attracts circulating neutrophils into the injury site. VPN inhibits TNF-α induced-IKKα/β activation with reduction of target genes activations and reduction of various forms of proinflammatory cytokines and mediator following I/R injury in IS, **Figure 3** [35, 36].

In addition, injured neurons in IS release specific proteins called danger associated molecular patterns including; heat shock protein (HSP), high mobility group-box 1 protein (HMGB-1), ATP and nicotinamide adenine dinucleotide (NAD) which activate TLR4 receptors on perivascular macrophage, microglia and endothelial cells. Therefore, TLR4 antagonist reduces infarct size attenuates IS-induced inflammatory changes and I/R injury [37, 38]. Different in *vitro* and in *vivo* studies illustrated that VPN inhibits I/R injury in IS through suppression of TLR4 receptors and NF-$_{K}$B signaling pathway in animal model studies [39].

Neuronal mitochondrial reactive oxygen species (ROS) contribute into the pathogenesis of I/R injury in IS as well as neurodegeneration and glutamate excitotoxicity [40]. VPN activates peripheral benzodiazepine receptors (BBRs) which regulate mitochondrial outer cell membrane and prevent the opening of mitochondrial permeability transition pore (MPTP). Furthermore, VPN prevents mitochondrial dysfunction through the prevention of mitochondrial depolarization, inhibition of mitochondrial Na^{+}/Ca^{2+} exchange, prevention of mitochondrial Ca^{+2} release, MPTP opening and the release of free radicals from outer mitochondrial membrane during neuronal injury [41]. Therefore, VPN regulates mitochondrial redox homeostasis through induction of ATP hydrolysis, inhibition of mitochondrial respiration and regulation of ATP synthesis. Thus, VPN preserves mitochondrial integrity and attenuates inflammatory and oxidative damage following I/R injury in IS. Moreover, Qiu et al., illustrated that VPN is effective in reducing the volume of cerebral infarct and

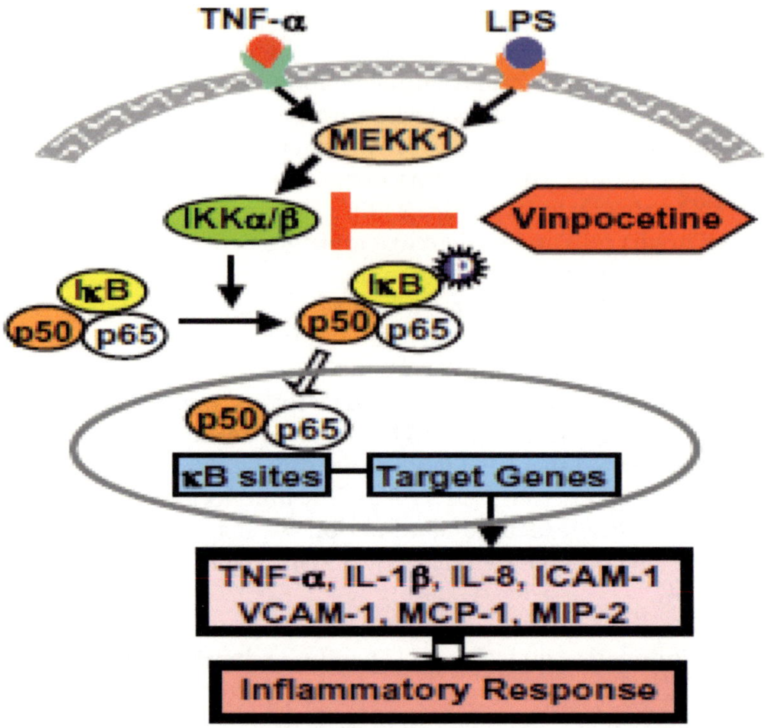

Figure 3.
Effects of vinpocetine on proinflammatory mediators during ischemic-reperfusion (I/R) injury in ischemic stroke.

attenuation I/R injury through down-regulation of NF-KB p65 and cyclo-oxygenase 2(COX-2) with up-regulation of peroxisome proliferator-activator receptor γ(PPARγ) which is neuroprotective mediator during IS [42].

3.4 Vinpocetine and post-ischemic stroke

3.4.1 Immunological and inflammatory reactions in post-ischemic stroke

In the brain, there is multiple communications between glial cell and other immune cells, which together participate in the immune reactions during ischemic events. In the post-ischemic stroke (PIS), B-cell, T-cell, macrophage and neutrophils enter the brain to connect and engage glial cells in immune interactions. This interaction maintains homeostasis and prevents further neuronal damage through generation of pro-survival factors like transforming growth factor-β and IL-10 which promote the resolution of inflammations [43].

It has been noticed, that IS activates neuro-inflammations which increase the permeability of BBB leading to activation of mast cells and macrophages which release histamine and pro-inflammatory cytokines respectively which recruit immune cell to the site of injury leading to progression of ischemic injury [44].

Therefore, the relationship between immune cells and neurons during IS is so intricate relationship.

Microglia is regarded as a first line defense mechanism of innate immunity against ischemic injury which activated within hours following IS. There are two activation pathways for microglia, which are classical pathway (M1) and alternative pathway (M2). M1 activation leads to induction of inducible nitric oxide synthase

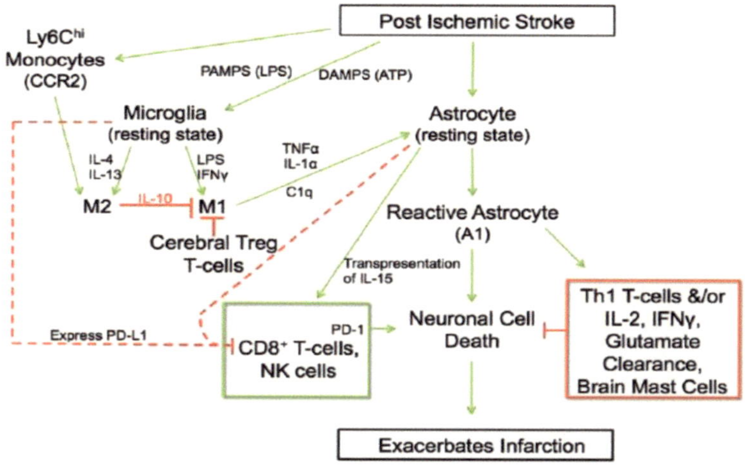

Figure 4.
Microglial and astrocyte activations in post-ischemic stroke. CCR2: chemokine receptor 2; PAMPs: pathogen-associated molecular patterns; LPS: lipopolysaccharides; PD-1: programmed death-ligand 1; NK: natural killer; CD: cluster of differentiation.

(iNOS) and TNF-α causing neuronal damage while; M2 activation leads to induction the release of pro-inflammatory cytokines and arginase leading to neuroprotection [45]. Aging is associated with impaired M2 activation and thus; M1 activation overriding M2 causing more inflammatory changes in elderly patients with IS [46].

Similarly, astrocyte which is another type of glial cell contributes in the formation of BBB and activated following IS. Reactive astrocyte subdivided into A1plays a role in the neuronal damage through upregulation of complement genes, and A2 plays a role in the neuroprotection through up-regulation of neurotrophic factors [47]. One month following PIS, astrocyte undergoes morphological and functional changes leading to reactive gliosis and activation of T-cell at ischemic regions [48].

Therefore, astrocyte and glial cells act as bridge interaction between neurons and immune system through different pro-inflammatory cytokines, **Figure 4** [49]. It has been shown that inflammatory changes, glial and astrocyte activations at post-stroke period participating together in the induction of different PIS complications such as depression, epilepsy, dementia and cognitive dysfunctions [50]. Vardian study illustrated that VPN have noteworthy antioxidant, anti-inflammatory and anti-apoptotic effects with inhibitory effect on glial and astrocyte cells during and following IS. Also, VPN reduces astrocyte edema and excitability through cAMP dependent-PKA pathway [51].

3.4.2 Vinpocetin for post-ischemic stroke epilepsy

Kim et al. reported that PIS predisposes for early and late onset epilepsy which called post-stroke seizure (PSS) due to the disturbances in the neuronal metabolic homeostasis, reactive gliosis, glutamate release and neuronal hyper-excitability [52]. Recently, Garza-Morales et al., found that VPN is effective as an adjuvant therapy in the management of epilepsy, it reduces seizure frequency by 50% in a dose of 2 mg/kg/day as compared with placebo [53]. The anti-epileptic mechanisms of VPN are through blockade of presynaptic Na-channels mediated glutamate release, inhibition of TNF-α and IL-1β which play a role in the augmentation of presynaptic Ca and Na permeability [54, 55].

3.4.3 Vinpocetin for post-stroke depression

Post-stroke depression (PSD) is a critical psychiatric complication of IS characterized by psychomotor disturbances, fatigue and sleep disorders with a prevalence of 33% following IS [56]. PSD is developed due to inflammatory reactions induced-neuroplasticity and imbalance of pro-inflammatory/anti-inflammatory ratio which causing glutamate excitotoxicity and intracellular Ca dysregulation [57]. Different studies illustrated that inflammatory cytokines induced-PSD lead to a reduction in the synthesis of serotonin, brain derived neurotrophic factor and fibroblast growth factor-2 which are important in the regulation of mood and neurotransmission [58, 59].

Inflammatory cytokines are implicated in the induction of PSD through activation of indolamine-2,3-dioxygenase at the marginal zone of the infracted area leading to depletion of serotonin and initiation of depression [60]. Furthermore, Wierner et al. found that nerve growth factor (NGF) which important secretory protein inhibits apoptosis and improves neuronal differentiations was low in PSD [61]. On the other hand, calcitonin gene-related peptide (CGRP) which is a neuroprotective peptide is elevated in patients with PSD and thus; CGRP antagonist could improve depressive symptoms [62].

Therefore, anti-inflammatory drugs with rehabilitation therapy enhance neuronal plasticity and functional recovery after IS [63]. VPN reduces the inflammatory processes and improves neuronal plasticity through inhibition the releases of inflammatory cytokines and chemokines from macrophage, microglia, and vascular smooth and endothelial cells with restoration of synaptic neurotransmissions [64]. As well, VPN improves psychomotor performances through modulation of brain monoamine pathway mainly on dopamine and serotonin, which play an integral role in attenuation of depressive symptoms [65]. Chen et al. reported that VPN improves neuronal functions and neurotransmission through modulation of NGF levels following IS [66]. Similarly, VPN improves neuronal transmission and inhibits induced pain pathway in PSD through down-regulation of CGRP [67]. Herewith, VPN attenuates PSD through different pathways either directly by activation of neuronal cAMP/cGMP pathway or indirectly through anti-oxidant, anti-inflammatory and modulation of brain peptides and neurotransmitters. Since, hippocampal cAMP-PKA response element of BDNF signaling pathway is decreased in patients with PSD. So, improvement of neuronal cAMP could interestingly prevent PSD [68].

3.4.4 Vinpocetin for post-stroke cognitive deficit

Post-stroke cognitive deficit (PSCD) is defined as global cognitive disability within 6 months after stroke regardless of presumptive causes according to American Psychiatric Associations Diagnostic and Statistical Manual of Mental Disorder. As well, 30% of stroke survivor found to have a noteworthy degree of cognitive decline within the first month after the stroke [69]. It has been noticed that some cognitive disorders may also develop subsequent to transient ischemic attack (TIA) suggesting that PSCD used in this way does not propose underlying neuro-pathological changes. Therefore, PSCD seems to be suitable for dementia, which associated with vascular insult and neuro-degenerative processes [70]. Various cross-sectional and longitudinal studies illustrated a link between high levels of inflammatory biomarkers in stroke survivors and risk of PSCD. Erythrocyte sedimentation rate (ESR), C-reactive protein (CRP), IL-12 and IL-6 sera levels are elevated in patients with PSD and regarded as predictor factors [71, 72].

The inflammatory mechanism of PSCD is related to the dysregulation in inflammatory and immune factors since; reduction of IL-8 and IL-6 are associated with changes in both white and gray matters, suggesting a role in the pathogenesis of

PSCD. As well, IL-1, IL-10, TNF-α and α-synuclien are increased in PSCD [73]. Shen and Gao study reported that high somatostatin and low neuron specific enolase in patients with PSCD compared to the healthy controls [74].

Other mechanisms of PSCD are cerebral hypoperfusion, reduction in cerebrovascular reserve capacity, impairment of cerebral vasoreactivity and autoregulatory ability which together initiate abnormal neuronal cell membrane phosphorylation and amyloid beta formation [75]. In addition, irreversibly injured astrocytes are converted to clasmatodendrosis which leads to disruption of gliovascular association at BBB in the white matter. Clasmatodendrosis is associated with cognitive disorders in patients with PSCD [76]. From these points, the mechanisms of PSCD remain obscure due to overlapping between neuro-pathological data and findings of PSCD and Alzheimer disease [77]. VPN improves cognitive functions and spatial memory through inhibition of hippocampal and cortical PDE-1with augmentation of cAMP/cGMP ratio, enhancement of cholinergic neurotransmission and inhibition of neuronal IKK/NF-kB [78, 79]. It has been noticed by Bitner study that both cAMP and cGMP activate PKA and cAMP-response element-binding protein (CREP) which improves synaptic plasticity and neurogenesis through up-regulation of BDNF. cAMP/cGMP/CREP pathway increases early and late long-term potentiation of memory [80] Besides, other PDE inhibitors like sildenafil (PDE-5 inhibitors) and cilostazol (PDE-3 inhibitor) also improve cognitive function and PSCD [81]. Recently, McQuown et al. illustrated that VPN improves memory function mainly through inhibition of PDE-1B isoform as it mainly located in regions with high dopaminergic neurotransmission such as the prefrontal cortex, striatum and dentate gyrus [78]. Therefore, VPN is an effective therapy in rehabilitation of cognitive, memory deficit and PSCD through modulation of inflammatory changes and enhancement of neuronal cAMP/cGMP in post-stroke survivors [82].

4. Conclusions

VPN is an effective agent in the management of ischemic stroke and plays an integral role in the prevention and attenuation of post-stroke epilepsy, depression and cognitive deficit through direct cAMP/cGMP-dependent pathway or indirectly through anti-inflammatory and anti-oxidant effects.

Author details

Hayder M. Al-kuraishy* and Ali I. Al-Gareeb
Department of Pharmacology, Toxicology and Medicine College of Medicine
Al-Mustansiriya University, Iraq, Baghdad

*Address all correspondence to: hayderm36@yahoo.com

References

[1] Alkuraishy HM, Al-Gareeb AI, Albuhadilly AK. Vinpocetine and pyritinol: A new model for blood rheological modulation in cerebrovascular disorders a randomized controlled clinical study. BioMed Research International. 2014;**2014**:1-8

[2] El-Laithy HM, Shoukry O, Mahran LG. Novel sugar esters proniosomes for transdermal delivery of vinpocetine: Preclinical and clinical studies. European Journal of Pharmaceutics and Biopharmaceutics. 2011;**77**(1):43-55

[3] Cao B, Ding Q, Liu X, Liu C, Songhua HU. Clinical observation of sofren injection combined with vinpocetine injection in the treatment of acute massive cerebral infarction. China Pharmacy. 2017;**28**(32):4527-4529

[4] Nadeem RI. Evaluation of the possible neurobehavioral effects of vinpocetine in parkinsonian-like models in rats [CU Theses]; 2018

[5] Zhang F, Yan C, Wei C, Yao Y, Ma X, Gong Z, et al. Vinpocetine inhibits NF-κB-dependent inflammation in acute ischemic stroke patients. Translational Stroke Research. 2018;**9**(2):174-184

[6] Manda V, Avula B, Dale O, Chittiboyina A, Khan I, Walker L, et al. Studies on pharmacokinetic drug interaction potential of vinpocetine. Medicine. 2015;**2**(2):93-105

[7] Cerami C, Perani D. Imaging neuroinflammation in ischemic stroke and in the atherosclerotic vascular disease. Current Vascular Pharmacology. 2015;**13**(2):218-222

[8] Arboix A. Cardiovascular risk factors for acute stroke: Risk profiles in the different subtypes of ischemic stroke. World Journal of Clinical Cases. 2015;**3**(5):418

[9] Go AS, Mozaffarian D, Roger VL, Benjamin EJ, Berry JD, Borden WB, et al. Executive summary: Heart disease and stroke statistics—2013 update: A report from the American Heart Association. Circulation. 2013;**127**(1):143-152

[10] Macrez R, Ali C, Toutirais O, Le Mauff B, Defer G, Dirnagl U, et al. Stroke and the immune system: From pathophysiology to new therapeutic strategies. The Lancet Neurology. 2011;**10**(5):471-480

[11] Sidorov E, Sanghera DK, Vanamala JK. Biomarker for ischemic stroke using metabolome: A clinician perspective. Journal of Stroke. 2019;**21**(1):31

[12] Yang C, Hawkins KE, Doré S, Candelario-Jalil E. Neuroinflammatory mechanisms of blood-brain barrier damage in ischemic stroke. American Journal of Physiology-Cell Physiology. 2018;**316**(2):C135-C153

[13] Zarruk JG, Greenhalgh AD, David S. Microglia and macrophages differ in their inflammatory profile after permanent brain ischemia. Experimental Neurology. 2018;**301**:120-132

[14] Wu LR, Liu L, Xiong XY, Zhang Q, Wang FX, Gong CX, et al. Vinpocetine alleviate cerebral ischemia/reperfusion injury by down-regulating TLR4/MyD88/NF-κB signaling. Oncotarget. 2017;**8**(46):80315

[15] Fujita M, Imaizumi M, Zoghbi SS, Fujimura Y, Farris AG, Suhara T, et al. Kinetic analysis in healthy humans of a novel positron emission tomography radioligand to image the peripheral

benzodiazepine receptor, a potential biomarker for inflammation. NeuroImage. 2008;**40**(1):43-52

[16] Svab G, Doczi J, Gerencser AA, Ambrus A, Gallyas F, Sümegi B, et al. The mitochondrial targets of neuroprotective drug vinpocetine on primary neuron cultures, brain capillary endothelial cells, synaptosomes, and brain mitochondria. Neurochemical Research. 2019;**18**:1-3

[17] Patyar S, Prakash A, Modi M, Medhi B. Role of vinpocetine in cerebrovascular diseases. Pharmacological Reports. 2011;**63**(3):618-628

[18] Ahmed HI, Abdel-Sattar SA, Zaky HS. Vinpocetine halts ketamine-induced schizophrenia-like deficits in rats: Impact on BDNF and GSK-3β/β-catenin pathway. Naunyn-Schmiedeberg's Archives of Pharmacology. 2018;**391**(12):1327-1338

[19] Zhang W, Huang Y, Li Y, Tan L, Nao J, Hu H, et al. Efficacy and safety of vinpocetine as part of treatment for acute cerebral infarction: A randomized, open-label, controlled, multicenter CAVIN (Chinese assessment for vinpocetine in neurology) trial. Clinical Drug Investigation. 2016;**36**(9):697-704

[20] Jack C. Interventions that may increase cerebral blood flow. In: Alzheimer's Turning Point. Cham: Springer; 2016. pp. 217-228

[21] Slemmer JE, Shacka JJ, Sweeney MI, Weber JT. Antioxidants and free radical scavengers for the treatment of stroke, traumatic brain injury and aging. Current Medicinal Chemistry. 2008;**15**(4):404-414

[22] Al-Kuraishy HM, Al-Gareeb AI, Al-Nami MS. Vinpocetine improves oxidative stress and pro-inflammatory mediators in acute kidney injury. International Journal of Preventive Medicine. 2019;**10**:1-6

[23] Santos MS, Duarte AI, Moreira PI, Oliveira CR. Synaptosomal response to oxidative stress: Effect of vinpocetine. Free Radical Research. 2000;**32**(1):57-66

[24] Abdel-Salam OM, Khadrawy YA, Salem NA, Sleem AA. Oxidative stress in a model of toxic demyelination in rat brain: The effect of piracetam and vinpocetine. Neurochemical Research. 2011;**36**(6):1062-1072

[25] Abdel-Salam OM, Hamdy SM, Seadawy SA, Galal AF, Abouelfadl DM, Atrees SS. Effect of piracetam, vincamine, vinpocetine, and donepezil on oxidative stress and neurodegeneration induced by aluminum chloride in rats. Comparative Clinical Pathology. 2016;**25**(2):305-318

[26] Deshmukh R, Sharma V, Mehan S, Sharma N, Bedi KL. Amelioration of intracerebroventricular streptozotocin induced cognitive dysfunction and oxidative stress by vinpocetine—A PDE1 inhibitor. European Journal of Pharmacology. 2009;**620**(1-3):49-56

[27] Ishola IO, Akinyede AA, Adeluwa TP, Micah C. Novel action of vinpocetine in the prevention of paraquat-induced parkinsonism in mice: Involvement of oxidative stress and neuroinflammation. Metabolic Brain Disease. 2018;**33**(5):1493-1500

[28] Gao W, Xiong Y, Li Q, Yang H. Inhibition of toll-like receptor signaling as a promising therapy for inflammatory diseases: A journey from molecular to nano therapeutics. Frontiers in Physiology. 2017;**8**:508

[29] Zhang L, Yang L. Anti-inflammatory effects of vinpocetine in atherosclerosis and ischemic stroke: A review of the literature. Molecules. 2015;**20**(1):335-347

[30] Cohen PA. Vinpocetine: An unapproved drug sold as a dietary supplement. In: Mayo Clinic Proceedings. Elsevier; 2015;**90**(10):1455

[31] Medina AE. Vinpocetine as a potent antiinflammatory agent. Proceedings of the National Academy of Sciences. 2010;**107**(22):9921-9922

[32] Ma Y, Wang J, Wang Y, Yang GY. The biphasic function of microglia in ischemic stroke. Progress in Neurobiology. 2017;**157**:247-272

[33] Zhao YY, Yu JZ, Li QY, Ma CG, Lu CZ, Xiao BG. TSPO-specific ligand vinpocetine exerts a neuroprotective effect by suppressing microglial inflammation. Neuron Glia Biology. 2011;7(2-4):187-197

[34] Wang H, Zhang K, Zhao L, Tang J, Gao L, Wei Z. Anti-inflammatory effects of vinpocetine on the functional expression of nuclear factor-kappa B and tumor necrosis factor-alpha in a rat model of cerebral ischemia–reperfusion injury. Neuroscience Letters. 2014;**566**:247-251

[35] Jeon KI, Xu X, Aizawa T, Lim JH, Jono H, Kwon DS, et al. Vinpocetine inhibits NF-κB–dependent inflammation via an IKK-dependent but PDE-independent mechanism. Proceedings of the National Academy of Sciences. 2010;**107**(21):9795-9800

[36] Nivison-Smith L, Khoo P, Acosta ML, Kalloniatis M. Pre-treatment with vinpocetine protects against retinal ischemia. Experimental Eye Research. 2017;**154**:126-138

[37] Abdel-Rahman EA, Mahmoud AM, Aaliya A, Radwan Y, Yasseen B, Al-Okda A, et al. Resolving contributions of oxygen-consuming and ROS-generating enzymes at the synapse. Oxidative Medicine and Cellular Longevity. 2016;**2016**:1-7

[38] Valencia A, Sapp E, Kimm JS, McClory H, Reeves PB, Alexander J, et al. Elevated NADPH oxidase activity contributes to oxidative stress and cell death in Huntington's disease. Human Molecular Genetics. 2013;**22**(6):1112

[39] Essam RM, Ahmed LA, Abdelsalam RM, El-Khatib AS. Phosphodiestrase-1 and 4 inhibitors ameliorate liver fibrosis in rats: Modulation of cAMP/CREB/TLR4 inflammatory and fibrogenic pathways. Life Sciences. 2019;**222**:245-254

[40] Colombo BB, Fattori V, Guazelli CF, Zaninelli TH, Carvalho TT, Ferraz CR, et al. Vinpocetine ameliorates acetic acid-induced colitis by inhibiting NF-κB activation in mice. Inflammation. 2018;**41**(4):1276-1289

[41] Nag S, Krasikova R, Airaksinen AJ, Arakawa R, Petukhovd M, Gulyas B. Synthesis and biological evaluation of [18F] fluorovinpocetine, a potential PET radioligand for TSPO imaging. Bioorganic & Medicinal Chemistry Letters. 2019;**20**:2270-2274

[42] Qiu X, Wang J, Lanying HE, Luo Y. Vinpocetine alleviates cerebral ischemia-reperfusion injury in rats by regulation of the expressions of nuclear factor κB p65, peroxisome proliferator-activated receptor γ and cyclooxygenase-2. International Journal of Cerebrovascular Disease and Stroke. 2015;**23**(7):517-521

[43] Yan J, Greer JM, Etherington K, Cadigan GP, Cavanagh H, Henderson RD, et al. Immune activation in the peripheral blood of patients with acute ischemic stroke. Journal of Neuroimmunology. 2009;**206**(1-2):112-117

[44] Lambertsen KL, Finsen B, Clausen BH. Post-stroke inflammation—Target or tool for therapy? Acta Neuropathologica. 2019;**137**(5):693-714

[45] Xu L, He D, Bai Y. Microglia-mediated inflammation and neurodegenerative disease. Molecular Neurobiology. 2016;**53**(10):6709-6715

[46] Lee DC, Ruiz CR, Lebson L, Selenica ML, Rizer J, Hunt JB Jr, et al. Aging enhances classical activation but mitigates alternative activation in the central nervous system. Neurobiology of Aging. 2013;**34**(6):1610-1620

[47] Liu Z, Chopp M. Astrocytes, therapeutic targets for neuroprotection and neurorestoration in ischemic stroke. Progress in Neurobiology. 2016;**144**:103-120

[48] Pekny M, Wilhelmsson U, Tatlisumak T, Pekna M. Astrocyte activation and reactive gliosis—A new target in stroke? Neuroscience Letters. 2019;**689**:45-55

[49] Hersh J, Yang SH. Glia–immune interactions post-ischemic stroke and potential therapies. Experimental Biology and Medicine. 2018;**243**(17-18):1302-1312

[50] Ahangar AA, Saadat P, Alijanpour S, Galeshi M, Hosseinalipour S. Post ischemic stroke complication: How much nursing diagnosis are confirms by neurologist. Journal of Patient Care. 2018;**4**(140):2

[51] Vardjan N. Mechanism and drug targets for reducing cell edema (neuroprotection) and cytoplasmic excitability in astrocytes in normal and pathological states. United States patent US 9,970,924; 2018. p. 15

[52] Kim HJ, Park KD, Choi KG, Lee HW. Clinical predictors of seizure recurrence after the first post-ischemic stroke seizure (vol. 16, p. 212, 2016). BMC Neurology. 2017;**17**:1-9

[53] Garza-Morales S, Briceño-González E, Ceja-Moreno H, Ruiz-Sandoval JL, Góngora-Rivera F, Rodríguez-Leyva I, et al. Extended-release vinpocetine: A possible adjuvant treatment for focal onset epileptic seizures. Boletín Médico del Hospital Infantil de México. 2019;**76**(5):215-224

[54] Sitges M, Sanchez-Tafolla BM, Chiu LM, Aldana BI, Guarneros A. Vinpocetine inhibits glutamate release induced by the convulsive agent 4-aminopyridine more potently than several antiepileptic drugs. Epilepsy Research. 2011;**96**(3):257-266

[55] Gómez CD, Buijs RM, Sitges M. The anti-seizure drugs vinpocetine and carbamazepine, but not valproic acid, reduce inflammatory IL-1β and TNF-α expression in rat hippocampus. Journal of Neurochemistry. 2014;**130**(6):770-779

[56] Llorca GE, Castilla-Guerra L, Moreno MF, Doblado SR, Hernández MJ. Post-stroke depression: An update. Neurología. 2015;**30**(1):23-31

[57] Levada OA, Troyan AS. Poststroke depression biomarkers: A narrative review. Frontiers in Neurology. 2018;**9**:577-586

[58] Pascoe MC, Crewther SG, Carey LM, Crewther DP. Inflammation and depression: Why poststroke depression may be the norm and not the exception. International Journal of Stroke. 2011;**6**(2):128-135

[59] Anisman H, Hayley S. Inflammatory factors contribute to depression and its comorbid conditions. Science Signaling. 2012;**5**(244):pe45

[60] Spalletta G, Bossu P, Ciaramella A, Bria P, Caltagirone C, Robinson RG. The etiology of poststroke depression: A review of the literature and a new hypothesis involving inflammatory cytokines. Molecular Psychiatry. 2006;**11**(11):984

[61] Wiener CD, de Mello Ferreira S, Moreira FP, Bittencourt G, de Oliveira JF,

Molina ML, et al. Serum levels of nerve growth factor (NGF) in patients with major depression disorder and suicide risk. Journal of Affective Disorders. 2015;**184**:245-248

[62] Shao B, Zhou YL, Wang H, Lin YS. The role of calcitonin gene-related peptide in post-stroke depression in chronic mild stress-treated ischemic rats. Physiology & Behavior. 2015;**139**:224-230

[63] Greifzu F, Schmidt S, Schmidt KF, Kreikemeier K, Witte OW, Löwel S. Global impairment and therapeutic restoration of visual plasticity mechanisms after a localized cortical stroke. Proceedings of the National Academy of Sciences. 2011;**108**(37):15450-15455

[64] Lourenco-Gonzalez Y, Fattori V, Domiciano TP, Rossaneis AC, Borghi SM, Zaninelli TH, et al. Repurposing of the nootropic drug Vinpocetine as an analgesic and anti-inflammatory agent: Evidence in a mouse model of superoxide anion-triggered inflammation. Mediators of Inflammation. 2019;**2019**:1-9

[65] Al-Gareeb AI, Al-Windy S, Al-Kuraishy H. The effects of vinpocetine on the psychomotor performances: Randomized clinical trial, single blind random clinical study. Al-Nahrain Journal of Science. 2012;**15**(3):129-133

[66] Chen Q, Li GQ, Li JT. Effect of ganglioside combined with vinpocetine therapy on neural functional reconstruction in convalescents with acute cerebral infarction. Journal of Hainan Medical University. 2016;**22**(22):27-30

[67] Csillik B, Mihály A, Knyihár-Csillik E. Antinociceptive effect of vinpocetine--a comprehensive survey. Ideggyógyászati Szemle. 2010;**63**(5-6):185-192

[68] Wang C, Guo J, Guo R. Effect of XingPiJieYu decoction on spatial learning and memory and cAMP-PKA-CREB-BDNF pathway in rat model of depression through chronic unpredictable stress. BMC Complementary and Alternative Medicine. 2017;**17**(1):73

[69] Henon H, Durieu I, Guerouaou D, Lebert F, Pasquier F, Leys D. Poststroke dementia: Incidence and relationship to prestroke cognitive decline. Neurology. 2001;**57**(7):1216-1222

[70] Justin BN, Turek M, Hakim AM. Heart disease as a risk factor for dementia. Clinical Epidemiology. 2013;**5**:135

[71] Rothenburg LS, Herrmann N, Swardfager W, Black SE, Tennen G, Kiss A, et al. The relationship between inflammatory markers and post stroke cognitive impairment. Journal of Geriatric Psychiatry and Neurology. 2010;**23**(3):199-205

[72] Narasimhalu K, Lee J, Leong YL, Ma L, De Silva DA, Wong MC, et al. Inflammatory markers and their association with post stroke cognitive decline. International Journal of Stroke. 2015;**10**(4):513-518

[73] Jokinen H, Melkas S, Ylikoski R, Pohjasvaara T, Kaste M, Erkinjuntti T, et al. Post-stroke cognitive impairment is common even after successful clinical recovery. European Journal of Neurology. 2015;**22**(9):1288-1294

[74] Shen Y, Gao HM. Serum somatostatin and neuron-specific enolase might be biochemical markers of vascular dementia in the early stage. International Journal of Clinical and Experimental Medicine. 2015;**8**(10):19471

[75] Hagberg G, Fure B, Thommessen B, Ihle-Hansen H, Øksengård AR, Nygård S, et al. Predictors for favorable cognitive

outcome post-stroke: A-seven-year follow-up study. Dementia and Geriatric Cognitive Disorders. 2019;**28**:1-1

[76] Hase Y, Horsburgh K, Ihara M, Kalaria RN. White matter degeneration in vascular and other ageing-related dementias. Journal of Neurochemistry. 2018;**144**(5):617-633

[77] Akinyemi RO, Allan LM, Oakley A, Kalaria RN. Hippocampal neurodegenerative pathology in post-stroke dementia compared to other dementias and aging controls. Frontiers in Neuroscience. 2017;**11**:717

[78] McQuown S, Xia S, Baumgärtel K, Barido R, Anderson G, Dyck B, et al. Phosphodiesterase 1b (PDE1B) regulates spatial and contextual memory in hippocampus. Frontiers in Molecular Neuroscience. 2019;**12**:21-33

[79] Ali AA, Ahmed HI, Khaleel SA, Abu-Elfotuh K. Vinpocetine mitigates aluminum-induced cognitive impairment in socially isolated rats. Physiology & Behavior. 2019;**1**:112571-112586

[80] Bitner RS. Cyclic AMP response element-binding protein (CREB) phosphorylation: A mechanistic marker in the development of memory enhancing Alzheimer's disease therapeutics. Biochemical Pharmacology. 2012;**83**(6):705-714

[81] Reneerkens OA, Rutten K, Steinbusch HW, Blokland A, Prickaerts J. Selective phosphodiesterase inhibitors: A promising target for cognition enhancement. Psychopharmacology. 2009;**202**(1-3):419-443

[82] Jacquin A, Binquet C, Rouaud O, Graule-Petot A, Daubail B, Osseby GV, et al. Post-stroke cognitive impairment: high prevalence and determining factors in a cohort of mild stroke. Journal of Alzheimer's Disease. 2014;**40**(4):1029-1038